Curbside
Consultation
in Hip Arthroplasty

49 Clinical Questions

CURBSIDE CONSULTATION IN ORTHOPEDICS
SERIES

SERIES EDITOR, BERNARD R. BACH, JR., MD

Curbside Consultation
in Hip Arthroplasty

49 Clinical Questions

EDITED BY

SCOTT M. SPORER, MD

MIDWEST ORTHOPAEDICS AT RUSH

CHICAGO, ILLINOIS

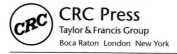

CRC Press
Taylor & Francis Group
Boca Raton London New York

CRC Press is an imprint of the
Taylor & Francis Group, an **informa** business

First published 2008 by SLACK Incorporated

Published 2024 by CRC Press
2385 NW Executive Center Drive, Suite 320, Boca Raton FL 33431

and by CRC Press
4 Park Square, Milton Park, Abingdon, Oxon, OX14 4RN

CRC Press is an imprint of Taylor & Francis Group, LLC

Library of Congress Cataloging-in-Publication Data

Curbside consultation in hip arthroplasty : 49 clinical questions / [edited by] Scott Sporer.
    p. ; cm. -- (Curbside consultation in orthopedics)
  Includes bibliographical references and index.
  ISBN 978-1-55642-830-2 (alk. paper)
  1. Arthroplasty--Miscellanea. I. Sporer, Scott. II. Series.
  [DNLM: 1. Arthroplasty, Replacement, Hip. 2. Hip Joint--surgery. WE 860 C975 2008]
  RD686.C87 2008
  617.5'810592--dc22
                          2008022496

ISBN: 9781556428302 (pbk)
ISBN: 9781003523550 (ebk)

DOI: 10.1201/9781003523550

Dedication

This book is dedicated to my wife, Alissa, who has sacrificed so much so that I could pursue my dreams.

Contents

About the Editor

Scott M. Sporer, MD is an orthopaedic total joint replacement surgeon in Chicago and holds an academic appointment at the rank of Assistant Professor at RUSH University Medical Center. He attended medical school at The University of Iowa before completing his orthopaedic residency training at Dartmouth Hitchcock Medical Center. He has completed a fellowship in adult reconstruction at RUSH Medical Center and currently has a clinical practice focusing on hip and knee arthroplasty. Dr. Sporer has a strong interest in clinical outcomes research and has completed a master's program at Dartmouth College in the evaluative clinical sciences.

Contributing Authors

Michael Archibeck, MD (Question 36)
New Mexico Center for Joint Replacement
Surgery
New Mexico Orthopaedics
Albuquerque, NM

William V. Arnold, MD, PhD (Question 45)
Orthopaedic Surgeon and Clinical
Instructor
Rothman Institute of Orthopaedics
Jefferson Medical College
Philadelphia, PA

Jorge Aziz-Jacobo, MD (Question 3)
International Research Fellow
Joint Implant Surgeons, Inc
New Albany, OH
International Research Fellow
Plano Orthopaedics and Sports Medicine
Center
Plano, TX

J. Todd Bagwell, MD (Question 42)
Board Certified Internal Medicine/Infec-
tious Disease
Austin Infectious Disease Consultants
Austin, TX

Robert L. Barrack, MD (Question 43)
Charles and Joanne Knight Distinguished
Professor of Orthopedic Surgery
Washington University Department of
Orthopaedic Surgery
Chief of Staff for Orthopedic Surgery
Barnes-Jewish Hospital
St. Louis, MO

Matthew Beal, MD (Question 20)
Orthopaedic Surgery Resident Physician
University of Chicago Medical Center
Chicago, IL

Paul E. Beaulé, MD, FRCSC (Question 26)
Associate Professor
Head of Adult Reconstruction, The Ottawa
Hospital
University of Ottawa
Ottawa, Ontario, Canada

Keith R. Berend, MD (Question 3)
Associate
Joint Implant Surgeons, Inc
Clinical Assistant Professor
Department of Orthopaedics
The Ohio State University
Attending Surgeon
Mount Carmel Health System
New Albany, OH

Michael E. Berend, MD (Question 33)
Center for Hip and Knee Surgery
Fellowship Director, Joint Replacement
Surgeons of Indiana Research Foundation
Volunteer Clinical Professor, Indiana
University School of Medicine
Indianapolis, IN

Thomas E. Brown, MD (Question 6)
Associate Professor
Department of Orthopaedic Surgery
University of Virginia
Charlottesville, VA

R. Stephen J. Burnett, MD, FRCS(C)
(Question 43)
Division of Orthopaedic Surgery
University of British Columbia
Island Medical Program—Royal Jubilee
Hospital
Victoria, British Columbia, Canada

Charles R. Clark, MD (Question 37)
Dr. Michael Bonfiglio Professor of Ortho-
paedics and Rehabilitation
Carver College of Medicine
Professor of Biomedical Engineering
College of Engineering
University of Iowa
Iowa City, IA

Quan Jun Cui, MD (Question 6)
Assistant Professor
Department of Orthopaedic Surgery
University of Virginia
Charlottesville, VA

Marc M. DeHart, MD (Question 39)
Clinical Assistant Professor
Department of Orthopaedic Surgery and
Rehabilitation
University of Texas Medical Branch
Adult Hip and Knee Reconstruction,
Texas Orthopedics, Sports & Rehabilitation
Associates
Austin, TX

Carl Deirmengian, MD (Question 7)
Booth Bartolozzi Balderston Orthopaedics
Philadelphia, PA
Lankenau Hospital
Wynnewood, PA

Craig J. Della Valle, MD (Question 38)
Midwest Orthopedics at RUSH
Chicago, IL

Paul E. Di Cesare, MD (Question 5)
Chair, Department of Orthopaedic
Surgery
UC Davis Medical Center
Sacramento, CA

Mark Dumonski, MD (Question 49)
Rush University Medical Center
Chicago, IL

Thomas K. Fehring, MD (Question 24)
OrthoCarolina Hip & Knee Center
Charlotte, NC

Kevin B. Fricka, MD (Question 41)
The Anderson Orthopaedic Clinic
Alexandria, VA

Donald S. Garbuz, MD, FRCSC (Question 44)
Associate Professor and Head
Division of Lower Limb Reconstruction
and Oncology
Department of Orthopaedics
University of British Columbia
Vancouver, British Columbia, Canada

Tad L. Gerlinger, MD (Question 48)
Program Director, Orthopaedic Surgery
Residency Chief, Adult Reconstruction
Brooke   Army   Medical   Center
Fort Sam Houston, TX

Raju S. Ghate, MD (Question 16)
Northwestern University
Feinberg School of Medicine
Chicago, IL

Andrew H. Glassman, MD, MS (Question 30)
Attending Physician
Grant Medical Center
Associate Clinical Professor of Orthopaedic
Surgery
The Ohio State University
Columbus, OH

Devon D. Goetz, MD (Question 46)
Des Moines Orthopaedic Surgeons
West Des Moines, IA
Associate Professor
Clinical Department of Orthopaedic
Surgery
University of Iowa Hospitals and Clinics
Iowa City, IA

Allan E. Gross, MD, FRCSC, OOnt
(Question 11)
Professor, Department of Surgery
Mt. Sinai Hospital
University of Toronto
Toronto, Ontario, Canada

William G. Hamilton, MD (Question 34)
Anderson Orthopaedic Institute
Alexandria, VA

William J. Hozack, MD (Question 45)
Professor of Orthopedic Surgery
Director, Joint Replacement Service
Thomas Jefferson University
Philadelphia, PA

Richard Illgen II, MD (Question 2)
Co-Director of the University of Wisconsin
Joint Replacement Program
The University of Wisconsin Medical School
Madison, WI

Duncan Jacks, MD (Question 14)
Department of Orthopaedics
University of British Columbia
Vancouver, British Columbia, Canada

Kenneth D. Kleist, MD (Question 47)
Adjunct Assistant Professor
University of Minnesota
HealthPartners Medical Group
Regions Hospital
St. Paul, MN

Brett Levine, MD, MS (Question 21)
Assistant Professor
Rush University Medical Center
Chicago, IL

William A. Lighthart, MD (Question 32)
Vermont Orthopaedic Clinic
Rutland Regional Medical Center
Rutland, VT

Saul Magitsky, MD (Question 12)
Sturdy Memorial Hospital
Attleboro, MA

David Manning, MD (Question 20)
Assistant Professor of Surgery
Section of Orthopaedic Surgery
Director of Arthroplasty Service
University of Chicago Medical Center
Chicago, IL

Amanda D. Marshall, MD (Question 13)
Department of Orthopaedics
University of Texas Health Science Center
San Antonio, TX

John L. Masonis, MD (Question 24)
OrthoCarolina Hip & Knee Center
Charlotte, NC

Bassam A. Masri, MD, FRCSC (Question 14)
Professor and Chairman
Department of Orthopaedics
University of British Columbia
Vancouver, British Columbia, Canada

R. Michael Meneghini, MD
(Questions 8 and 35)
New England Musculoskeletal Institute
University of Connecticut Health Center
Farmington, CT

William Mihalko, MD, PhD (Question 6)
Associate Professor
Department of Orthopaedic Surgery
University of Virginia
Charlottesville, VA

Calin S. Moucha, MD (Question 19)
Chief, Division of Joint Replacement &
Reconstruction
North Jersey Orthopaedic Institute
Assistant Professor
Department of Orthopaedics
New Jersey Medical School
University of Medicine & Dentistry of New
Jersey
Newark, NJ

Brian P. Murphy, MD, MS (Question 17)
Bloomington Bone and Joint Arthritis
Institute
Bloomington, IN

Steve Mussett, MD, FRCSC (Question 26)
Fellow, Adult Reconstruction
University of Ottawa
Ottawa, Ontario, Canada

Steven Ogden, MD (Question 29)
Texas Hip and Knee Center
Fort Worth, TX

Kirstina Olson, MD (Question 20)
Orthopaedic Surgery Resident Physician
University of Chicago Medical Center
Chicago, IL

Michael O'Rourke, MD (Question 28)
Illinois Bone and Joint Institute, LLC
Director, Total Joint Replacement Center
Evanston Northwestern Healthcare
Glenview, IL

Hari Parvataneni, MD (Question 27)
Assistant Professor
Department of Orthopaedic Surgery
University of Miami
Miami, FL

Jeffrey L. Pierson, MD (Questions 8 and 35)
St. Vincent Center for Joint Replacement
Indianapolis, IN

Harry E. Rubash, MD (Question 27)
Chief of Orthopaedic Surgery
Massachusetts General Hospital
Edith M. Ashley Professor of Orthopaedic
Surgery
Harvard Medical School
Boston, MA

James A. Ryan, MD (Question 5)
Adult Reconstruction Fellow
Hospital for Special Surgery
New York, NY

Khaled Saleh, MD, FRCSC (Question 6)
Professor
Department of Orthopaedic Surgery
University of Virginia
Charlottesville, VA

Mark F. Schinsky, MD (Question 23)
Castle Orthopaedics & Sports Medicine,
SC
Aurora, IL

W. Randall Schultz, MD, MS (Question 42)
Board Certified Orthopedic Surgeon
The Orthopedic Group
Austin, TX

Todd Sekundiak, MD, FRCS (Question 31)
Department of Orthopaedic Surgery
Creighton University Medical Center
Omaha, NE

*Alexander Siegmeth, MD, FRCS
(Questions 14 and 44)*
Consultant Orthopaedic Surgeon
Department of Orthopaedics
Golden Jubilee National Hospital
Glasgow, United Kingdom

James Slover, MD, MS (Question 18)
NYU Hospital for Joint Diseases
New York, NY

Vivek Sood, MD (Question 4)
Midwest Orthopaedics at RUSH
Chicago, IL

Matthew W. Squire, MD, MS (Question 2)
Assistant Professor
Department of Orthopedics and Rehabilitation
University of Wisconsin Hospitals and Clinics
Madison, WI

Michael J. Taunton, MD (Question 10)
Mayo Clinic
Rochester, MN

Robert T. Trousdale, MD (Question 10)
Mayo Clinic
Rochester, MN

Walter W. Virkus, MD (Question 49)
Rush University Medical Center
Cook County Hospital
Chicago, IL

Stephen M. Walsh, MD, FRCSC (Question 22)
DownEast Orthopedic Associates, PA
Bangor, ME
Eastern Maine Medical Center
Bangor, ME
St. Joseph Hospital
Bangor, ME

Steven H. Weeden, MD (Question 29)
Fellowship Director
Texas Hip and Knee Center
Fort Worth, TX

Preface

Orthopaedic surgeons are faced daily with difficult clinical situations. A consultation with a colleague can provide great insight into various treatment options and alternatives to maximize patient outcomes. *Curbside Consultation in Hip Arthroplasty* allows the reader the opportunity to "consult" an expert in the field of total hip arthroplasty and obtain a clinically relevant suggestion for patient care rather than reviewing a lengthy text without clinically relevant solutions.

Introduction

Curbside Consultation in Hip Arthroplasty is a unique text that was written for residents, fellows, and practicing orthopaedic surgeons who encounter difficult clinical situations surrounding total hip replacement. This book was written by a group of surgeons with expertise in the field of primary and revision total hip arthroplasty. Forty-nine common clinical scenarios are discussed, with each scenario resulting in a brief "consultation" with an expert that will provide practical and clinically relevant information. The unique Q&A format provides quick access to current information related to hip arthroplasty with the simplicity of a conversation between two colleagues. The text is intended to help answer the question we ask so frequently, "What would you do with a guy that has..."

SECTION I

PREOPERATIVE
GENERAL QUESTIONS

I Have a 43-Year-Old Male Who Needs a Total Hip Arthroplasty. Should I Use Highly Cross-Linked Polyethylene, Ceramic, or a Metal-on-Metal Bearing Surface?

Scott M. Sporer, MD

Patients undergoing total joint replacement today are often different than patients who had undergone joint replacement in the past. Today, total hip arthroplasty is considered an option for the younger and more active patient with end-stage hip arthritis. The demands this patient population places upon its articulation are distinctly different than in the past due to the relatively long service life, increased activity, and the desire of these patients to return to a high functional level. Articular surface wear with associated osteolysis is a cause of hip replacement failure and is more common in young, active patients. Newer articulations such as cross-linked polyethylene, ceramics-on-ceramic bearing surfaces, and metal-on-metal bearing surfaces have been introduced with the goal of minimizing volumetric wear and reducing the number of biologically active particles. The goal of each of these "alternative bearings" is to reduce the wear to a level that will not incite clinically significant osteolysis or cause the need for early revision.

Figure 1-1. Five-year follow-up of a primary total hip arthroplasty using a cobalt-chrome head against a highly cross-linked polyethylene liner. Note no associated osteolysis or demonstrable polyethylene wear.

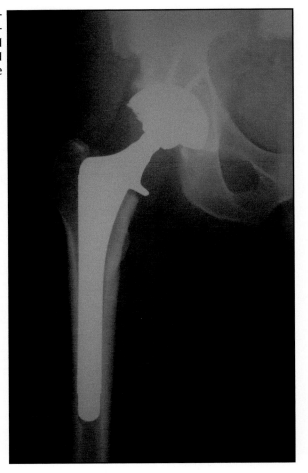

Ultra high molecular weight polyethylene has been the preferred bearing surface for many years. This material has shown few systemic complications and has minimal chance of acute catastrophic failure. However, this material is limited by its wear characteristics. Cross-linking is a method used to improve the wear resistance of polyethylene by forming a covalent bond between free radicals within the polyethylene. Cross-linking has been shown in hip simulators to markedly reduce the wear commonly seen in hip replacement by greater than 95% (Figure 1-1). Early clinical studies would support the claims of reduced wear but would suggest wear reductions closer to 60% to 70% as compared to conventional polyethylene. Unfortunately, cross-linking does affect the mechanical properties of the polyethylene, resulting in decreased yield strength, tensile strength, and elongation to failure. Clinically, the decrease in mechanical strength has not been a problem unless the acetabular component has been malpositioned and the polyethylene is subjected to nonphysiologic stress. The manufacturing process of the currently available cross-linked polyethylene components varies. The final sterilization may be different depending upon the manufacturer, the type and dose of irradiation used to cause the cross-linking, the subsequent thermal stabilization, and the machining. As a result, not all polyethylene liners should be considered equivalent and each particular material should be evaluated separately. The concern with all bearing surfaces is the wear particles' ability to incite a biologic reaction with resulting osteolysis. Substantial differences have been observed between cross-linked and non–cross-linked polyethylene liners in vitro. It appears that the particles released in cross-linked polyethylene are smaller and are less bioreactive. Additionally, the volumetric wear rates in hip simulators have been shown to be less with a larger diameter femoral head in appropriately positioned components. A larger diameter femoral head will provide a greater arc of motion before impingement and may minimize the risk of dislocation. Another option to reduce wear with a cross-linked polyethylene liner is to utilize a ceramic femoral head. Ceramics provide a decreased surface roughness and have been shown to result in a 50% reduction in wear. Concerns for ceramic heads include potential for catastrophic fracture, limited head and neck sizes, and increase in cost. While in vitro studies are encouraging for the use of cross-linked polyethylene liners, longer clinical follow-up is required before this bearing surface is universally recommended.

Metal-on-metal bearings have a long clinical record and were initially introduced as an alternative bearing surface to metal-on-polyethylene. Some metal-on-metal designs experienced early failures and as a result were abandoned. However, at longer follow-up, the survivorship of a metal-on-metal hip is comparable with a Charnley metal-on-polyethylene implant. Well-functioning metal-on-metal implants have been shown to have up to a 200 time reduction in volumetric wear rates compared to conventional polyethylene. The subtle design and manufacturing differences in metal-on-metal articulations appears crucial to the long-term results. The diameter of the acetabular shell in relation to the femoral head, the surface roughness, and the lubrication of the bearing can result in substantial differences in wear rates. Fluid film lubrication is the goal of a metal-on-metal articulation. In order to achieve this, the femoral head should be made as large as possible, the clearance between the cup and head should be as small as possible, and the surfaces should have a very low surface roughness. Wrought materials also appear to have better wear characteristics than forged implants. A metal-on-metal bearing encourages the use of a larger femoral head, which will improve the arc of motion before component-component impingement occurs and can potentially minimize the risk of instability (Figure 1-2). Acetabular component positioning is critical with a metal-on-metal articulation since component impingement between the cup and trunion can result in high levels of metal debris. The wear particles produced with a metal-on-metal articulation are substantially smaller than those associated with more conventional articulations. Despite the marked reduction in volumetric wear, the number of particles produced with a metal-on-metal articulation has been shown to be up to 500 times the number produced with a metal-on-polyethylene articulation. The significance of this larger number of particles and associated larger surface area is unknown. Elevated metal ion concentrations of both cobalt and chromium have been observed in the serum, erythrocytes, and urine in patients with these articulations. These elevated levels within the body have raised concern for delayed hypersensitivity reactions and progression of renal failure, along with concern for carcinogenesis. Most studies to date have failed to establish a correlation between elevated metal ion concentration and elevated cancer risk. However, ongoing evaluation is crucial since the latency period of several carcinogens is several years. Elevated metal ion concentrations have also been observed in fetal blood. As a result, a metal-on-metal articulation is not recommended for women of childbearing age or individuals with renal failure or risk factors of developing future renal failure.

Figure 1-2. Surface replacement with a metal-on-metal articulation. Note that a large femoral head provides improved wear characteristics and minimizes the chance of dislocation.

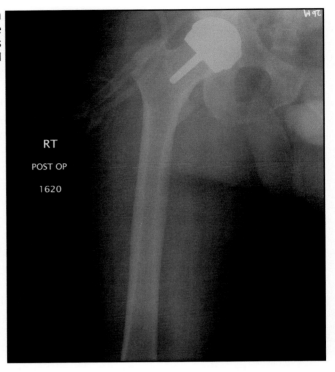

RT

POST OP

1620

Ceramic-on-ceramic bearings were introduced to provide an alternative bearing surface with low wear rates while avoiding some of the potential complications associated with metal bearings. Ceramics have been shown in vivo to produce the lowest volumetric wear rates due to the hydrophobic properties of ceramics along with their ability to be polished to a very smooth surface. Early ceramic designs were flawed in their manufacturing process and resulted in an unacceptable rate of fracture. Current generation ceramics are made from alumina and possess the optimal characteristics of low porosity, high density, and a small grain size. Ceramic-on-ceramic bearings require meticulous surgical technique both to avoid chipping of the liner during insertion and to place both the acetabular and femoral components in the appropriate anatomic position. Failure to place the implants in the correct position has led to early failure of the acetabular liner due to impingement. While the volumetric wear rates of ceramic bearings in vivo are less than that of either metal-on-polyethylene or metal-on-metal, ceramic articulations demonstrate a bimodal distribution of particle size, including both submicron particles and those of size similar to polyethylene. Ceramic wear debris is not bio inert as once thought and can induce osteolysis in some designs. While the early clinical results of current generation ceramic-on-ceramic bearings are encouraging, this bearing couple does have some limitations. Modular ceramic femoral head sizes are limited due to the strength required at the junction to avoid fracture. Consequently, the intraoperative flexibility to adjust leg length may be limited. Similarly, revision surgery may be complicated due to fewer options regarding the femoral head size and length. Recently, there has been a growing concern about "squeaking" of the ceramic articulation. This has been shown to occur in up to 7% of patients receiving these articulations.

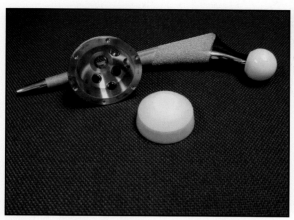

Figure 1-3. Ceramic-on-ceramic bearing. Note the need to insert the ceramic liner into the titanium shell. Care must be taken during insertion to avoid "chipping" the liner.

My current practice is to use a cobalt-chrome femoral head and a cross-linked polyethylene liner for the vast majority of patients requiring a total hip arthroplasty. Early in vivo data appear to correlate very closely with the in vitro lab data. Polyethylene has been shown to be a very durable bearing surface without the concerns for systemic illness. I have abandoned the use of a ceramic articulation due to the concerns of squeaking, the limited intraoperative options, failure of randomized clinical trials to demonstrate improved survival rates, and the necessity for "perfect" component placement. As surgeons we all strive to obtain a "perfect" result in every patient, but unfortunately, even with the use of surgical navigation, component position and orientation remain variable. Unlike polyethylene, ceramic-on-ceramic articulations are not forgiving and will result in early failure with subtle component malposition (Figure 1-3). Also, while the prevalence of ceramic femoral head fracture is minimal, this complication remains catastrophic when it occurs. I do continue to use metal-on-metal articulations in a subset of young patients. I believe this bearing is advantageous in patients who are employed in manual labor that requires them to work above ground or in a location that places the hip at a risk for dislocation (eg, carpenter, steel worker). I generally do not use this bearing in patients over the age of 55 since the results of a large-diameter metal-on-cross-linked polyethylene liner appear promising. I continue to avoid the use of metal-on-metal articulations in patients with a known metal hypersensitivity, women of childbearing age, and in patients who are at risk of developing renal failure.

Bibliography

Greenwald G. Alternative bearing surfaces: the good, the bad, and the ugly. *J Bone Joint Surg Am.* 2001;83: S68–S72.

Heisel C, Silva M, Schmalzried TP. Bearing surface options for total hip replacement in young patients. *Instr Course Lect.* 2004;53:49-65.

Jarrett CA, Ranawat A, Bruzzone M, Rodriguez J, Ranawat C. The squeaking hip: an underreported phenomenon of ceramic-on-ceramic total hip arthroplasty. *J Arthroplasty.* 2007;22(2):302.

I Have a Patient With Both Back and Hip Arthritis. How Do I Determine Which Is Most Problematic and Causing the Patient's Symptoms?

Matthew W. Squire, MD, MS
Richard Illgen II, MD

Coexistence of spine and hip pathology is common and can present significant diagnostic and therapeutic challenges to the orthopedic clinician. As with most orthopedic conditions, a basic understanding of anatomy, thorough patient history, appropriate physical examination, and plain radiographic examination of the hip and spine will frequently allow the adult reconstructive surgeon to determine the most likely etiology of the patient's pain. Unfortunately, patients who present with radiographic evidence of both hip arthritis and lumbar spine pathology often have buttock, lateral hip, or proximal thigh pain that is not easily ascribed to either the hip or spine.

The classic presentation of hip arthritis is groin pain either at rest or with activity that is reproduced by hip flexion and internal rotation. The clinical presentation of spine pathology is somewhat more variable and may be manifested by lower lumbar or sacroiliac pain, radiculopathy with pain below the knee, and/or neurogenic claudication. The femoral nerve stretch test (Figure 2-1) is an important provocative maneuver for patients with combined hip and spine pathology, as it can detect the presence of an irritated femoral nerve, which contains the nerve root responsible for innervating the hip capsule (L3).

Orthogonal plain radiographs should be the starting point for examination of the hip and lumbar spine, as they can easily detect significant hip arthritis as well as many types of lumbar spine pathology. However, judicious use of more advanced imaging can at times be helpful to the clinician. When warranted by cues in the history (corticosteroid use or alcohol abuse) and physical examination (positive test for labral pathology), hip magnetic resonance imaging (MRI) combined with intra-articular gadolinium (MRI arthrogram) can occasionally detect symptomatic hip pathology such as early femoral head

Figure 2-1. Femoral nerve stretch test.

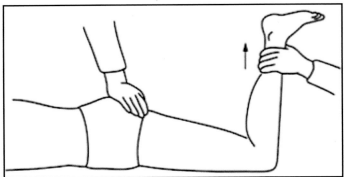

avascular necrosis or acetabular labral tears. In contrast, MRI examination of the lumbar spine frequently reveals pathologic changes that can either help (eg, severe stenosis with same-sided nerve root compression) or confuse (eg, mild stenosis and degenerative disc disease) the clinician in his or her quest to determine the etiology of the patient's pain.

When the clinician cannot confidently ascribe a patient's pain to either the hip or spine, use of the hip anesthetic arthrogram can correctly identify the etiology of the patient's pain and predict the pain relief a patient will have following a total hip arthroplasty (THA)[1] (Figure 2-2). Briefly, local anesthetic is injected into the hip joint under fluoroscopic guidance, and the patient's pain response is monitored either via a diary or having the patient return to clinic for re-examination 1 to 4 hours after the injection. Patients responding favorably (significant pain relief following anesthetic hip injection) were demonstrated to have excellent pain relief following THA in 20 of 21 patients. Patients who did not favorably respond to anesthetic hip injection for the most part responded well to nonoperative spine therapy, which improved symptoms in 7 of 8 patients. The positive and negative predictive values of hip anesthetic arthrogram in the above-mentioned study were 95% and 87%, respectively. Anesthetic hip injection showed a very low side effect profile (one vasovagal response) and was well tolerated by patients.

An alternative strategy to injecting the hip joint is injection of the spine. Selective nerve root blocks and/or epidural steroids may be offered depending on the pathology suspected or identified on physical examination and diagnostic imaging. Pain relief following injection would certainly support the suspicion that pathology within the lumbar spine is generating the patient's pain. However, failure to achieve pain relief following spine injection does not confirm the location of the pain generator and additional studies (eg, anesthetic arthrogram, sacroiliac [SI] joint injection) would be necessary to further define the etiology of the patient's pain. Currently, there is no evidence detailing the efficacy of diagnostic spine injection as a means to predict pain relief following THA in patients with concomitant hip arthritis and spine pathology.

At the author's institution, hip anesthetic arthrograms are performed for all patients with atypical hip pain where history, physical examination, and imaging studies are not sufficient to establish the diagnosis of symptomatic hip pathology warranting THA. Acceptance and tolerance of this approach are nearly universal, as the rationale and interpretation of this diagnostic test are easily understood by the vast majority of patients. To date, this approach has proven to be an extremely effective diagnostic strategy in patients with combined arthritis of the hip and spine as well as for patients with less common diagnoses.

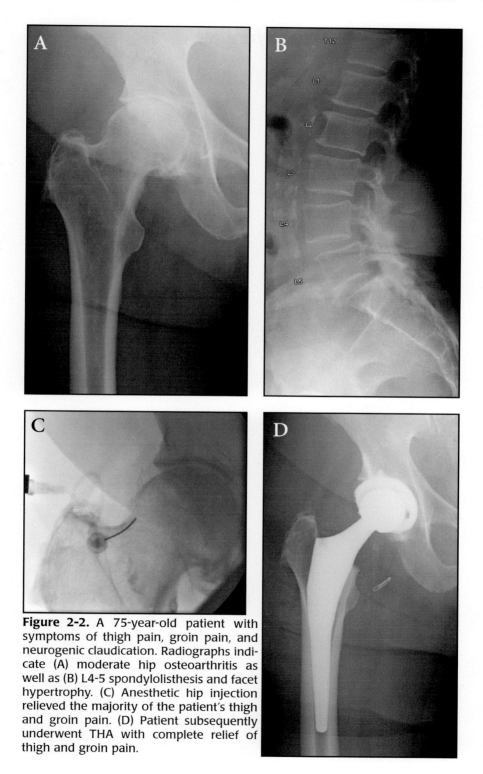

Figure 2-2. A 75-year-old patient with symptoms of thigh pain, groin pain, and neurogenic claudication. Radiographs indicate (A) moderate hip osteoarthritis as well as (B) L4-5 spondylolisthesis and facet hypertrophy. (C) Anesthetic hip injection relieved the majority of the patient's thigh and groin pain. (D) Patient subsequently underwent THA with complete relief of thigh and groin pain.

Reference

1. Illgen RL, Honkamp NJ, Weisman MH, Hagenauer ME, Heiner JP, Anderson PA. The diagnostic and predictive value of hip anesthetic arthrograms in selected patients before total hip arthroplasty. *J Arthroplasty*. 2006;21(5):724–730.

I HAVE A PATIENT WITH SEVERE BILATERAL HIP DEGENERATIVE ARTHRITIS. DO I PERFORM BILATERAL TOTAL HIP REPLACEMENT, OR DO I STAGE THE SURGERY? IF I DO STAGE THE SURGERY, HOW LONG SHOULD I WAIT?

Keith R. Berend, MD
Jorge Aziz-Jacobo, MD

Osteoarthritis of the hip presents as bilateral disease in up to 42% of patients.[1] The topic of simultaneous versus staged bilateral total hip arthroplasties (THA) continues to evoke controversy in the orthopaedic community. Perioperative complications represent the most significant issues.

Proponents of simultaneous bilateral THA cite the advantage of a one-anesthetic risk, a potentially shorter disability and recovery period, and reduced charges to hospital and patient.

We, however, would strongly recommend against a simultaneous procedure performed under a single anesthetic in favor of a two-stage approach. Routinely we would stage the procedures 6 weeks apart. The most important factor behind this recommendation is a reported significantly higher incidence of thromboembolic disease in the simultaneous group, which translates into a higher occurrence of pulmonary embolism.[2]

Moreover, the intraoperative blood loss is greater in the simultaneous group, even when compared with the combined loss during two-stage procedures. This is reflected in a significantly higher number of patients requiring allogeneic blood transfusions in the simultaneous group.[3–5] While transfusion is considered safe, the potential health risks associated with allogeneic blood include the transmission of blood-borne infections (such as those caused by the human immunodeficiency virus and hepatitis viruses), transfusion-related and allergic reactions, and immunomodulatory effects.[6] Despite the increased autologous and allogeneic transfusions, these bilateral simultaneous patients have a lower hemoglobin at discharge.[3] The functional recovery of these patients with anemia is likely to be adversely influenced and may increase length of hospital or rehabilitation stay.

We have systematically found that the patients with simultaneous THA do not reach their physical therapy goals for discharge to home during the hospital admission. While the cumulative length of stay for 2 admissions during staged procedures is longer, the simultaneous patients require significantly more inpatient rehabilitation services and thus incur increased costs. Due to the increased extent of the surgery, patients undergoing simultaneous bilateral procedures are more prone to minor complications such as postoperative ileus symptoms, electrolyte disturbances, mental status changes, and urinary tract infections.[4]

In a review at our institution of 227 consecutive patients undergoing either staged or simultaneous bilateral THA, all performed via an anterolateral approach with lateral decubitus positioning, the reoperation rate was significantly higher in the simultaneous group, with a wound complication/infection rate of 1.8% versus 0.5% (p = 0.01).[7] The dislocation rate was also significantly higher in the simultaneous group.[7] This may reflect patient positioning affecting acetabular orientation on the second side during surgery. Concern exists in relation to increased heterotopic ossification, reduced range of motion, and suboptimal gain in walking ability in patients undergoing simultaneous bilateral THA.[5]

We have systematically found that the patients with simultaneous THA do not reach their physical therapy goals for discharge to home during hospital admission and therefore require more inpatient rehabilitation services and increased costs.

Absolute contraindications for a simultaneous THA are patients with serious coexistent medical comorbidities or the elderly with obtunded physiologic compensatory mechanisms.[3] If you choose to perform simultaneous bilateral THA in a patient with bilateral disease, we strongly recommend that selection be limited to those patients having an American Society of Anesthesiology (ASA) score of 1 or 2, that thorough preoperative planning regarding blood supply be undertaken, and that extremely careful manipulation of the patient during change of position be realized. Furthermore, studies have suggested that preoperative evaluation by a qualified general medical consultant can identify patients who may be at increased risk. This preoperative evaluation can help in the final decision making.

If the procedure is done in a single anesthetic, there is no difference in the rate of deep or superficial infections among patients operated on with a different set or the same set of sterile instruments.[8]

While previous reports have noted a decreased cost with performing simultaneous procedures, these reports are skewed as they look only at hospital charges. This accounting falsely reduces cost to the hospital and ignores the actual reimbursement and increased burden to the health care system by transferring patients to skilled facilities and rehabilitation centers. Additionally, most surgeons are aware that the technical reimbursement for performing simultaneous bilateral THA is significantly less. This is despite an increased risk of complication and no reduction in the surgeon's overhead or liability.

While there are special cases when simultaneous bilateral THA makes sense, it is not the norm, and we would recommend staging the procedures 6 weeks apart. This provides the most cost-efficient paradigm for the hospital, surgeon, and health care system. Additionally, it is clearly safer in the majority of patients to proceed in 2 stages.

References

1. Tepper S, Hochberg MC. Factors associated with hip osteoarthritis: data from the First National Health and Nutrition Examination Survey (NHANES-I). *Am J Epidemiol.* 1993;137:1081-1088.
2. Berend ME, Ritter MA, Harty LD, et al. Simultaneous bilateral versus unilateral total hip arthroplasty: an outcome analysis. *J Arthroplasty.* 2005;20:421-426.
3. Parvizi J, Pour AE, Peak EL. One-stage bilateral total hip arthroplasty compared with unilateral total hip arthroplasty. *J Arthroplasty.* 2006;21(Suppl 6):26-31.
4. Swanson KC, Gonzales della Valle A, Salvati EA, et al. Perioperative morbidity after single-stage bilateral total hip arthroplasty: a matched control study. *Clin Orthop.* 2006;451:140-145.
5. Bhan S, Pankaj A, Malhotra R. One- or two-stage bilateral total hip arthroplasty: a prospective, randomized, controlled study in an Asian population. *J Bone Joint Surg.* 2006;88(3):298-303.
6. Bierbaum BE, Callaghan JJ, Galante JO, et al. An analysis of blood management in patients having a total hip or knee arthroplasty. *J Bone Joint Surg.* 2000;82(6):900-901.
7. Berend KR, Lombardi AV Jr, Adams JB. Simultaneous versus. staged cementless bilateral total hip arthroplasty: perioperative risk comparison. *J Arthroplasty.* 2007;22(6 Suppl):111-115.
8. Gonzales della Valle A, Walter WL, Peterson MG, et al. Prevalence of infection in bilateral total hip arthroplasty: A comparison of single-stage 565 bilateral procedures performed with 1 or 2 sets of instruments. *J Arthroplasty.* 2006;21:157-160.

How Do You Decide When a Patient Is "Ready" for a Total Hip Replacement? Is There a Downside to Waiting Until He or She Has More Severe Disease?

Vivek Sood, MD

When I see patients in the office for evaluation of hip pain, I start with a complete history and physical exam. Some important factors that I consider are the patient's age, limitations secondary to pain or stiffness, and his or her occupation. Once I determine that the pain is due to hip pathology and that the patient has failed conservative management (ie, lifestyle modification, weight loss, trial of different anti-inflammatory medications, and physical therapy), I have a discussion with the patient about total hip arthroplasty (THA). At this point, based on the patient's age, I explain what he or she can expect after a THA. Usually, patients over 60 have diminished physical activity at baseline, and they tend to have realistic expectations in terms of returning to baseline activity after surgery. In addition, their revision rate is low and acceptable. If the patient is between age 40 and 60, his or her activity level is still high. These patients tend to have high expectations postrecovery and will often need revisions, as they will wear out their implants (likely will need a bearing change/poly change). If the patient is younger than 40, his or her activity level is high, and life expectancy is another 30 to 40 years. This younger patient will likely need revision for implant wear (likely poly change with possibility of component revision). If the patient is very young (ie, in the second decade of life), I strongly recommend hip fusion as a bridging procedure, and 10 to 15 years later as he or she starts to develop back pain, contralateral hip pain, or ipsilateral knee pain, the hip fusion can be taken down and revised to a THA.

Despite the higher likelihood of future revisions in younger patients, the downside of waiting to undergo a THA is the patients can become severely limited in their activity because of pain and stiffness and can develop a worsening limp. According to a study by Garbuz et al, the odds of achieving a better-than-expected postoperative functional outcome decreased by 8% for each month that the patient delayed the hip surgery once THA was indicated.[1]

Twenty years ago, surgeons avoided doing THA on younger patients because of the bearing surface problems and because of a finite lifespan of cement. However, most THAs nowadays are done in press-fit fashion with biological fixation. Since biologic fixation has the potential to repair and remodel itself and the bearing surfaces have improved, surgeons today are pushing the age limitations by doing THA on younger patients.

Use of highly cross-linked poly or other hard bearing such as metal-on-metal or ceramics is allowing us to operate on younger patients. In addition, better locking mechanisms with modular poly allow us to change poly (relatively simpler revision) when wear is observed, further allowing us to push the age limits for THA. The use of highly cross-linked poly is still in its infancy, as we only have about 5-year follow-up studies.[2] However, early results clearly show lower wear rates and less osteolysis with highly cross-linked poly than with conventional poly. In a young male patient without renal problems, indicated for a THA, I would use metal-on-metal bearing surface after educating the patient about associated increase in metal ion levels.[3] I would avoid metal-on-metal in females of childbearing age. I do not use ceramic-on-ceramic in patients as a bearing surface, as this can lead to catastrophic failure due to ceramic fracture. In addition, there have been some reports of the squeaking phenomenon with the ceramic bearing surface. In recent literature, catastrophic failure because of ceramic fracture seems to be much less of an issue, but longer term follow-up is needed.

THA is an effective procedure with good long-term outcomes, and recent developments in surgical techniques and materials have allowed us to operate on younger patients.

References

1. Garbuz D, Xu M, Duncan C, Masri B, Sobolev B. Delays worsen quality of life outcome of primary total hip arthroplasty. *Clin Orthop Relat Res*. 2006;447:79–84.
2. Geerdink CH, Grimm B, Ramakrishnan R, Rondhuis J, Verburg AJ, Tonino AJ. Crosslinked polyethylene compared to conventional polyethylene in total hip replacement. *Acta Orthopaedica*. 2006;77(5):719–725.
3. MacDonald SJ, McCalden RW, Chess DG, et al. Metal-on-metal versus polyethylene in hip arthroplasty: a randomized clinical trial. *Clin Orthop Relat Res*. 2003;406:282–296.

I HAVE A 58-YEAR-OLD FEMALE ALCOHOLIC PATIENT WHO FELL AND HAS A FEMORAL NECK FRACTURE. WHAT SURGICAL APPROACH SHOULD I USE TO TREAT THIS FRACTURE, AND WHAT COMPONENT SHOULD I USE?

James A. Ryan, MD
Paul E. Di Cesare, MD

Background

Each year, approximately 350,000 US patients sustain a hip fracture, and this number is expected to double by 2050.[1] Hip fractures most commonly occur in elderly patients who sustain low-energy ground-level falls; they can also occur in younger patients with compromised bone quality or as a result of high-energy trauma. Orthopedic management decisions include type of operation, selection of implants, and surgical approach.

Type of Operation

Femoral neck fractures can be treated by open reduction with internal fixation, hemiarthroplasty, or total hip arthroplasty.[2] Issues to consider include patient factors (eg, premorbid hip pain, presence of arthritis, bone quality, premorbid medical conditions, functional status), fracture factors (eg, fracture pattern, level of comminution, fracture reducibility), and surgeon factors (eg, level of surgeon skill, experience performing a given procedure). While the chronological age of the current patient is 58 years, her physiologic age is likely much older. Her bone quality may be compromised given her history of alcoholism, and given that she exhibits 2 significant risk factors for osteonecrosis—alcoholism and femoral neck fracture—there is a strong possibility of late failure of internal fixation. For these reasons, the decision is made to proceed with total hip arthroplasty.

Selection of Implants

In choosing an implant, attention must be paid to specific complications for which a given patient is at risk. Alcoholism, history of fracture, and female gender are significant risk factors for postoperative dislocation.[3] Implant choice can be tailored to avoid this problem by using a large femoral head. We would choose to implant a 36-mm or greater femoral head, since larger femoral heads have been associated with decreased risk of dislocation due to improved head/neck ratio, increased "jump space" to dislocation, and decreased need for a skirted neck.[4] With a larger femoral head, attention must additionally be paid to an appropriate acetabular liner. Volumetric wear associated with a larger femoral head can be reduced with a liner of highly cross-linked polyethylene and/or an alternative bearing surface, such as ceramic-on-ceramic or metal-on-metal. In this patient we would prefer to implant a highly cross-linked polyethylene liner, as it would allow for reduced wear as well as allow a greater number of liner options (eg, elevated rim or lateralized liner) and would avoid the potential problem of elevated serum metal ions associated with the use of metal-on-metal implants. Although it has not been demonstrated that high levels of metal ions are associated with problems in healthy, active patients, this possibility cannot be so easily dismissed in an alcoholic patient with the potential for future hepatic and renal problems. A ceramic-on-ceramic bearing would be a reasonable option in this chronologically "young" patient if her anatomy can accommodate the limited ceramic liner/head options. We do not believe there is a role for primarily placing a constrained liner, even in a patient at higher risk for dislocation. We would use an in-growth acetabular cup placed via press-fit technique; such a system would allow for easy conversion to a constrained component if recurrent instability became a problem. The femoral stem options can be either cemented or uncemented; more recent studies support the use of proximally porous-coated, tapered stems, placed using a press-fit technique. Klein et al reported excellent bone ingrowth in 84 of 85 femoral stems utilizing this type of stem in elderly hip fracture patients, irrespective of bone quality.[5] In this case we would prefer to use a proximally porous-coated, tapered stem based on the patient's anatomy and bone quality, and we would be prepared to cement the stem if it were determined intraoperatively that the uncemented stem provided inadequate stability.

Surgical Approach

Given this patient's increased risk for postoperative dislocation, attention must be paid to the appropriate surgical approach. While there have been reports of higher dislocation rates following primary total hip arthroplasty via the posterolateral approach than other approaches, the use of larger femoral heads and improved capsular repair rates have decreased these rates substantially.[3] The anterolateral, direct lateral, or anterior approaches have been advocated by some as better options; however, patients may have a persistent limp. We believe surgeons should proceed with the approach with which they are most comfortable. In this case, we would proceed via the posterolateral approach, since we use this approach for primary total hip arthroplasty and believe that the larger femoral head in conjunction with posterior capsular repair results in a low risk of hip instability.

Conclusion

In proceeding with total hip arthroplasty in this patient, consideration must be given to her higher risk for dislocation. We would place implants and utilize the approach we use most commonly for our primary total hip arthroplasties, in particular by using a larger femoral head and a highly cross-linked polyethylene liner.

References

1. Morris AH, Zuckerman JD. National Consensus Conference on improving the continuum of care for patients with hip fracture. *J Bone Joint Surg Am.* 2002;84-A(4):670–674.
2. Macaulay W, Pagnatto MR, Iorio R, Mont MA, Saleh KJ. Displaced femoral neck fractures in the elderly: hemiarthroplasty versus total hip arthroplasty. *J Am Acad Orthop Surg.* 2006;14(5):287–293.
3. Soong M, Rubash HE, Macaulay W. Dislocation after total hip arthroplasty. *J Am Acad Orthop Surg.* 2004; 12(5):314–321.
4. Khatod M, Barber T, Paxton E, Namba R, Fithian D. An analysis of the risk of hip dislocation with a contemporary total joint registry. *Clin Orthop Relat Res.* 2006;447:19–23.
5. Klein GR, Parvizi J, Vegari DN, Rothman RH, Purtill JJ. Total hip arthroplasty for acute femoral neck fractures using a cementless tapered femoral stem. *J Arthroplasty.* 2006;21(8):1134–1140.

A 65-Year-Old Patient Fell and Has a Displaced Femoral Neck Fracture. Should I Do a Hemiarthroplasty or a Total Hip Arthroplasty?

Thomas E. Brown, MD
Khaled Saleh, MD, FRCSC
Quan Jun Cui, MD
William Mihalko, MD, PhD

For the treatment of displaced femoral neck fractures in physiologically older patients or for those greater than 65 years of age, it is generally accepted that replacement arthroplasty, when compared to open reduction and internal fixation, provides better functional results with fewer complications and lower reoperation rates.[1] The optimal type of arthroplasty to be performed (Austin-Moore, hemiarthroplasty, or total hip arthroplasty [THA]), however, has continued to generate considerable debate.

Historically, hemiarthroplasty for displaced fractures of the femoral neck has been the procedure of choice. The procedure is relatively quick and easy to perform with minimal assistance and has acceptably low short-term complication rates, including dislocation. Prosthesis options for hemiarthroplasty include mono-block, press-fit fracture stems, and modular unipolar or bipolar components. The decision as to implant choice and fixation technique (press-fit technique, polymethylmethacrylate [PMMA], or biologic fixation) is influenced by surgeon training and experience, patient age, bone quality, prefracture activity level, and implant cost, as well as the potential future need for revision or conversion to THA.

For many surgeons, THA has been utilized only for femoral neck fractures in patients with pre-existing arthritis because of the concern for arthritic groin pain and poor function postoperatively. THA has not been routinely utilized for fracture patients without pre-existing arthritis because of the surgeon's perceived good long-term function and pain relief achieved with hemiarthroplasty, as well as concerns for unacceptably high rates of dislocation postoperatively with THA.[2]

Two recent randomized controlled clinical trials directly comparing hemiarthroplasty and THA for displaced femoral neck fractures provide compelling evidence that function is better postoperatively with THA and that complication rates are comparable if not lower than for hemiarthroplasty. Additionally, the need for conversion surgery (hemi to THA) was higher than the need for revision THA surgery for any reason.[3,4]

Based on the available literature, if you are faced with treating a displaced femoral neck fracture, strong consideration should be given to performing an acute THA, unless severe infirmity, either physical or mental, places the patient at an increased risk of dislocation postoperatively. You can minimize the risk of dislocation by employing the following techniques:

* Consider the use of a surgical approach that involves an anterior capsulotomy (anterior, anterolateral, or direct lateral) to preserve the integrity of the posterior capsule. If a posterior approach is utilized, meticulous capsular repair is essential.

* Maximize the head:neck ratio of the prosthesis with the use of the largest head available. This will optimize impingement-free range of motion as well as the "jump distance" to further enhance stability.

* Extremely close attention must be paid to the position of both femoral and acetabular components, with rigorous intraoperative testing for stability in both anterior and posterior directions.

* Component fixation should be based on bone quality of the femur and acetabulum. Cemented fixation provides the surgeon with more flexibility in changing the version of the femoral component. Contrarily, cementless acetabular components provide the surgeon with more options with modular liners and easier reorientation of components, as dictated by intraoperative stability testing.

As mentioned previously, the decision to utilize a hemiarthroplasty for a displaced femoral neck fracture should be reserved for very elderly patients (>80 years old), institutionalized patients, walker-dependent patients, and those with significant cognitive impairment that would place them at an increased risk for dislocation. Fixation of the component should be durable and reliable (PMMA or biologic), and the component should be modular. Modularity allows for adequate restoration of the prefracture anatomy and also simplifies conversion to THA should the need arise. In the authors' opinion, bipolar hemiarthroplasty confers no advantages compared with modular unipolar devices and is an unnecessary expense. Additionally, closed reduction of a dislocated bipolar device may not be successful, necessitating another open procedure. Nonmodular press-fit devices should be reserved for minimal or nonambulatory patients, given the high incidence of component subsidence and pain for ambulatory patients.

With the impending epidemic of proximal femur fractures in the aging North American population, it is imperative that the orthopedic surgeon provide effective surgical treatment that is reliable, low risk, and reproducible and provides good long-term function for this ever-increasing segment of our society. For displaced femoral neck fractures, THA is the procedure of choice for the majority of ambulatory patients.

References

1. Bhandari M, Devereaux PJ, Swiontowski MF, et al. Internal fixation compared with arthroplasty for displaced fractures of the femoral neck: a meta-analysis. *J Bone Joint Surg Am.* 2003;85:1673–1681.
2. Papandrea RF, Froimson MI. Total hip arthroplasty after acute displaced femoral neck fractures. *Am J Orthop.* 1996;25:85–88.
3. Blomfeldt R, Tornkvist H, Eriksson K, et al. A randomized controlled trial comparing bipolar hemiarthroplasty with total hip replacement for displaced intracapsular fractures of the femoral neck in elderly patients. *J Bone Joint Surg Br.* 2007;2:160–165.
4. Baker RP, Squires B, Gargan MF, et al. Total hip arthroplasty and hemiarthroplasty in mobile, independent patients with a displaced intracapsular fracture of the femoral neck: a randomized controlled trial. *J Bone Joint Surg Am.* 2006;88:2583–2589.

I Have a 63-Year-Old Patient Who Is 6 Years Postoperative From a Total Hip Replacement. He Was Doing Very Well Until Last Week When He Began Experiencing Increasing Hip Pain Following a Dental Appointment. I Think His Hip Is Infected. What Should I Do?

Carl Deirmengian, MD

This patient should be seen immediately to expedite treatment. If this really is an acute infection, swift diagnosis and treatment are the keys to success. The first step is to rule out some common causes of hip pain. It is possible that the patient has sciatica or trochanteric bursitis, and an examination will aid in differentiating these etiologies of pain. The second step is a radiographic examination of the hip to evaluate the implant fixation and bony architecture. The physical exam and radiograph can be accomplished in one visit and will rule out infection for many patients. However, if the patient's symptoms cannot be firmly attributed to a known noninfectious etiology, then a workup for infection is necessary.

The algorithm for diagnosis of infection begins with laboratory tests, including the erythrocyte sedimentation rate (ESR), the C-reactive protein (CRP), and a peripheral blood count. The ESR and CRP are sensitive tests for infection, especially if both of these tests are elevated. The ESR and CRP are reasonably accurate tests for infection, especially when combined. If both are normal, the probability of infection is exceedingly low. If both are very high, there is very good evidence for infection. Intermediate or borderline results are more difficult to interpret, especially in the setting of inflammatory disease or other infections. The peripheral blood count is not a dependable test and cannot rule out infection, but elevations may indicate bacteremia.

If the suspicion of infection remains high, then a joint aspiration should be evaluated. Although not very useful for routine screening of painful hips, aspiration provides dependable results when utilized in select patients.[1] The aspiration allows culture for bacteria, as well as evaluation of the synovial fluid cell count. Preferably, the synovial fluid should be sent for cultures before antibiotics are started. A high cell count (synovial WBC >2500 with >60% PMN's) is very suggestive of infection, even in the absence of a positive culture. A low volume of fluid with a normal cell count and negative cultures would not be consistent with infection.

Usually, the clinical examination, history, radiographs, laboratory values, and aspiration lead to a clear diagnosis. However, there are situations when the diagnosis is still uncertain. In these cases, you may opt to obtain a bone scan, indium-labeled white blood cell (WBC) scan, or positron emission tomography (PET). Although the role of these imaging studies is not well defined, it appears that PET scanning has a good accuracy for diagnosing an infected hip arthroplasty.[2]

Acute hematogenous infections occur when bacteremia leads to an acutely infected implant. There are many sources of bacteremia, including ulcers, cellulitis, endocarditis, and cholecystitis among others. Additionally, procedures that cause bleeding in the mouth or foot are commonly thought to generate a transient bacteremia, with potential bacterial seeding of an arthroplasty. It is for this reason that prophylactic antibiotics are utilized.

When an arthroplasty patient becomes symptomatic with a presumed acute hematogenous infection, there is urgency to diagnose and treat. If an acute infection is diagnosed within 1 to 2 weeks, then the components may be retained, and there is a reasonable rate of success with irrigation and debridement with liner exchange.[3] Once an acute infection has been left untreated for more than 1 to 2 weeks, eradication will likely require removal of components. Although the reasons for this observation are not completely understood, it is generally thought that the bacteria are able to transform into the biofilm state, which is more resistant to treatment.

In contrast to acute hematogenous infections, chronic arthroplasty infections have a less dramatic presentation and are not generally associated with an identifiable cause. Patients may complain of months of increasing low-grade pain after a period of apparently normal postoperative function. In cases of chronic infection, without a recent clear bacterial source, it is generally accepted that removal of components is necessary for successful eradication.

The 63-year-old patient in this question is having sudden pain after a dental visit last week. This is a case of acute hematogenous infection, until proven otherwise, and there is urgency to the diagnosis. The rate of success for irrigation, debridement, and liner exchange is increased with prompt treatment. The key to decision making here is the diagnosis of infection to allow for appropriate treatment. If the examination, radiographs, ESR, CRP, and aspiration are consistent with infection, a prompt irrigation and debridement with liner exchange are indicated. Frozen section and multiple cultures should be sent intraoperatively to increase diagnostic accuracy. Postoperatively, the patient should be treated with 6 weeks of intravenous antibiotics.

References

1. Ali F, Wilkinson JM, Cooper JR, et al. Accuracy of joint aspiration for the preoperative diagnosis of infection in total hip arthroplasty. *J Arthroplasty*. 2006;21(2):221–226.
2. Pill SG, Parvizi J, Tang PH, et al. Comparison of fluorodeoxyglucose positron emission tomography and (111) indium-white blood cell imaging in the diagnosis of periprosthetic infection of the hip. *J Arthroplasty*. 2006;21(6 Suppl 2):91–97.
3. Marculescu CE, Berbari EF, Hanssen AD, et al. Outcome of prosthetic joint infections treated with debridement and retention of components. *Clin Infect Dis*. 2006; 42(4):471–478. Epub 2006 Jan 5.

SHOULD ALL OF MY PATIENTS DONATE BLOOD PRIOR TO TOTAL JOINT REPLACEMENT?

Jeffrey L. Pierson, MD
R. Michael Meneghini, MD

Major orthopedic surgery is associated with large amounts of blood loss, with a 46% reported rate of allogeneic and autologous transfusions in a large series of patients undergoing total joint arthroplasty (TJA). As such, orthopedic departments are typically large consumers of blood products within a hospital so the appropriate use of blood and blood-related resources should be a goal for orthopedic surgeons in their role as patient advocates and as stewards of the blood supply. For a variety of reasons, physicians and hospitals are developing multidisciplinary strategies to improve blood utilization, improve patient outcomes, and reduce costs (Tables 8-1 and 8-2). We define blood management as proactive processes, techniques, drugs, or medical devices that reduce the need for allogeneic blood when employed in an efficient, effective, and timely manner.

Blood utilization is suboptimal in many hospitals because of poor training and inadequate oversight, review, and monitoring of transfusion practices. The decision to administer blood is often clouded by myths, misconceptions, and emotions and not supported by good medical science. In spite of mounting evidence that demonstrates significant harm from unnecessary blood transfusions, there are several studies that document a generalized lack of compliance with appropriate transfusion guidelines, as well as tremendous variation in transfusion practice between different institutions and among individual physicians within the same institution.

Although the blood supply is the safest it has ever been, transfusion of blood components remains a high-risk procedure that results in some degree of harm to all patients. The benefits of transfusion therapy, however, especially the use of red cells, are not well elucidated. Few, if any, well-controlled studies demonstrate improved outcomes with red cells. The landmark TRICC trial published in 1999 involved a prospective randomized

Table 8-1
Orthopedic Blood Management Strategies

Preoperative

- Early identification of patients at high risk of transfusion
- Blood management algorithms
- Selective use of erythropoietic agents and iron therapy
- Discontinuation of drugs and herbal medicines that increase bleeding
- Autologous predonation (not recommended)

Intraoperative

- Minimization of surgical time
- Regional anesthesia
- Temperature maintenance
- Patient positioning
- Controlled "normotension"
- Cautery
- Topical hemostatic agents
- Intraoperative autotransfusion
- Antifibrinolytics (tranexamic acid, epsilon-aminocaproic acid) and serine protease inhibitors (aprotinin)
- Point of care testing
- Evidence-based transfusion decisions

Postoperative

- Evidence-based transfusion decisions
- Postoperative autotransfusion (washed)
- Minimize iatrogenic blood loss

Table 8-2
Blood Management Principles

- Early identification and intervention for patients at high risk for transfusions
- Utilization of current scientific evidence and the promotion of clinical best practices
- Alignment and coordination of all members of the health care team
- Patient advocacy and patient safety
- Stewardship of scarce and expensive hospital resources

trial of transfusion strategies in 838 intensive care unit patients. The authors' conclusion was that a restrictive strategy of red cell transfusions (Hgb 7.0) was at least as effective and possibly superior to a more liberal strategy (Hgb 9.0 to 10.0) with the possible exception of those patients with acute coronary syndromes. A study published in 2004 by cardiologists at Duke even questioned the benefit of transfusions in those high-risk cardiac populations. As with any medical therapy, the decision to transfuse must be made in the context of an informed risk and benefit analysis.

One of many concerns about predonation of autologous blood (PAB) is that the likelihood of any transfusion event is increased 7- to 12-fold in patients that predonate, increasing the risk of clerical error. Prolonged storage of blood products (up to 42 days for red blood cell) leads to a progressive decline in product quality and linear increases in debris and inflammatory mediators. These inflammatory mediators can result in systemic inflammatory syndrome (SIRS) and transfusion-related acute lung injury (TRALI). TRALI is the leading cause of transfusion-related morbidity and mortality worldwide and occurs with a frequency of 1:500 platelet transfusions and 1:1000 to 5000 plasma and red cell transfusions. Its occurrence is likely underreported because of a lack of awareness by clinicians.

Other problems with PAB include inconvenience, wastefulness (40% to 60% of units are discarded), the creation of a phlebotomy-induced anemia, and uncertainty regarding the indications for predonation by nonanemic patients.

Preoperative preparation and planning are essential elements for the safe and optimal management of surgical patients. Through the early identification of high-risk patients who are amenable to strategies to modify those risks, hospitals can improve patient outcomes and improve overall resource utilization through reduced adverse events.

Anemia management protocols are essential to blood management programs because they increase red cell mass in anemic patients, allowing them to reduce or eliminate their need for allogeneic blood during high blood loss surgeries. Paradoxically, the use of autologous predonated blood causes an iatrogenic anemia that is treated with a return of the predonated blood, without a net benefit to the patient. For this and other reasons detailed previously, we discourage the use of autologous predonation and endorse the use of algorithms that selectively employ preoperative erythropoietin (Figure 8-1). Our use of this algorithm for primary TJA has resulted in dramatic reductions in allogeneic blood transfusions. The incidence of allogeneic blood transfusions after primary total knee and hip arthroplasty is 1.4% and 2.8%, respectively.

As with intraoperative transfusion decisions, postoperative transfusions should be based upon measured lab values and using evidence-based protocols. Much of the symptomatology in postoperative orthopedic patients attributed to anemia is more causally related to volume deficits from postoperative bleeding, so aggressive but well-monitored volume replacement is generally sufficient to allow rehabilitation and timely discharge in patients with hemoglobins in the 7 to 8 g/dL range. As an aside, we feel that higher levels of hemoglobin in elderly patients are beneficial for rehabilitation potential, but we are not convinced that transfusing stored, allogeneic blood will improve their overall outcomes.

Conclusion

We recommend the use of a blood conservation algorithm for primary TJA that is characterized by discouraging the use of PAB, selective use of preoperative epoetin alfa, and the adoption of evidence-based transfusion criteria.

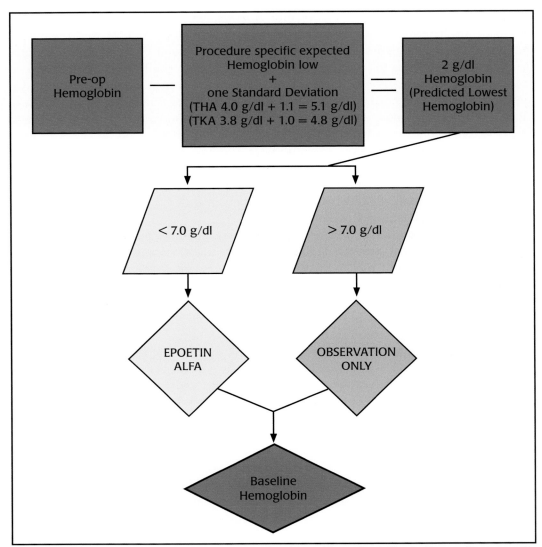

Figure 8-1. Orthopedic blood management algorithm. Flow chart illustrating patient specific recommendations. The preoperative hemoglobin is the hemoglobin before the patient enters the algorithm. The baseline hemoglobin is the hemoglobin at the time of surgery. (Adapted from Pierson JL, Hannon TJ, Earles DR. A blood-conservation algorithm to reduce blood transfusions after total hip and knee arthroplasty. *J Bone Joint Surg Am*. 2004;86-A:1512–1518.)

Bibliography

Bierbaum BE, Callaghan JJ, Galante JO, et al. An analysis of blood management in patients having a total hip or knee arthroplasty. *J Bone Joint Surg Am*. 1999;81:2-10.

Billote DB, Glisson SN, Green D, et al. A prospective, randomized study of preoperative autologous donation for hip replacement surgery. *J Bone Joint Surg Am*. 2002;84-A:1299-1304.

Buehler PW, Alayash AI. Toxicities of hemoglobin solutions: in search of in-vitro and in-vivo model systems. *Transfusion*. 2004;44:1516-1530.

Carson JL, Altman DG, Duff A, et al. Risk of bacterial infection associated with allogeneic blood transfusion among patients undergoing hip fracture repair. *Transfusion*. 1999;39:694-700.

Cremieux PY, Barrett B, Anderson K, et al. Cost of outpatient blood transfusion in cancer patients. *J Clin Oncol.* 2000;18:2755-2761.

Hansen E, Hansen MP. Reasons against the retransfusion of unwashed wound blood. *Transfusion.* 2004;44:45S-53S.

Hebert PC, Wells G, Blajchman MA, et al. A multicenter, randomized, controlled clinical trial of transfusion requirements in critical care. Transfusion Requirements in Critical Care Investigators, Canadian Critical Care Trials Group. *N Engl J Med.* 1999;340:409-417.

Keating EM, Meding JB. Perioperative blood management practices in elective orthopaedic surgery. *J Am Acad Orthop Surg.* 2002;10:393-400.

Parker MJ, Roberts CP, Hay D. Closed suction drainage for hip and knee arthroplasty: a meta-analysis. *J Bone Joint Surg Am.* 2004;86-A:1146-1152.

Pierson JL, Hannon TJ, Earles DR. A blood-conservation algorithm to reduce blood transfusions after total hip and knee arthroplasty. *J Bone Joint Surg Am.* 2004;86-A:1512-1518.

Poses RM, Berlin JA, Noveck H, et al. How you look determines what you find: severity of illness and variation in blood transfusion for hip fracture. *Am J Med.* 1998;105:198-206.

Rao SV, Jollis JG, Harrington RA, et al. Relationship of blood transfusion and clinical outcomes in patients with acute coronary syndromes. *JAMA.* 2004;292:1555-1562.

Spahn DR, Casutt M. Eliminating blood transfusions: new aspects and perspectives. *Anesthesiology.* 2000;93:242-255.

Spiess BD. Risks of transfusion: outcome focus. *Transfusion.* 2004;44:4S-14S.

Toy P, Popoversusky MA, Abraham E, et al. Transfusion-related acute lung injury: definition and review. *Crit Care Med.* 2005;33:721-726.

A 20-Year-Old Patient Suffered a Hip Dislocation in a Motor Vehicle Accident. He Has Developed Avascular Necrosis and Now Has Severe Degenerative Arthritis. How Do You Treat His Pain?

Scott M. Sporer, MD

Early hip arthritis in a young patient remains a challenging problem for joint replacement surgeons (Figure 9-1). Treatment options for very young patients with end-stage disease consist of delaying surgery, total hip replacement, resurfacing arthroplasty, hemiarthroplasty, femoral osteotomy, hip resection, or hip fusion. Each of these treatment modalities has perceived and realized advantages along with accompanying disadvantages. Increased rates of bearing surface wear, osteolysis, and aseptic loosening have been demonstrated in the younger, more active patient following total hip arthroplasty. The need for future revision surgery with the associated bone loss is a concern in patients expected to have 40 to 60 years of remaining life. Hip resurfacing is an attractive option for younger patients; however, poorer long-term results have been observed in patients with avascular necrosis.

Hemiarthroplasty has been shown to result in persistent pain, early component loosening, and loss of acetabular bone stock. Hip resection eliminates the potential for wear-induced osteolysis but results in a limb that is shortened, has decreased strength, and requires increased expenditure of energy for ambulation. Patients with a resection have significant limitations in their daily activities, and this option is considered unacceptable for most patients. Delaying surgical intervention in patients with end-stage arthritis

Figure 9-1. An 18-year-old male involved with unilateral post-traumatic osteoarthritis. Patient is employed in construction and had no clinical or radiographic evidence of low back, ipsilateral knee, or contralateral hip pain.

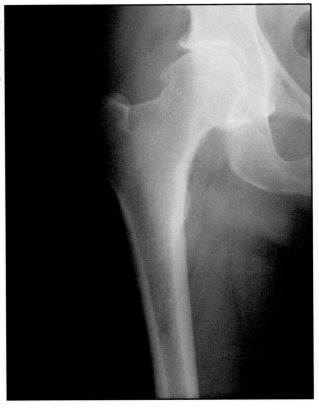

eliminates the concerns for bearing surface wear but requires patients to lead a more sedentary lifestyle. Patients with an arthritic hip also describe increased fatigue, weight gain, and decreased quality of life.

The treatment of severe hip arthritis in a young patient should alleviate current symptoms yet allow future surgical options. Total hip arthroplasty undoubtedly returns patients to a higher functional level with near immediate pain relief. However, failure rates of 30% to 40% have been observed in this cohort of patient at short- to mid-term follow-up. Male patients with unilateral hip disease requiring total hip replacement secondary to osteonecrosis or osteoarthritis appear to be at the greatest risk of early failure. Alternative bearing surfaces and newer implant designs are now available and may offer improved results. Despite these improvements, a service life of 40 to 60 years without revision is unlikely.

Hip arthrodesis remains an alternative for the treatment of severe hip arthritis. This option is considered less frequently today as the long-term outcomes of total hip arthroplasty improve. However, a well-performed arthrodesis can provide dramatic pain relief, allow patients to return to high-level activities, and can be converted to a successful total hip arthroplasty in the future. As with all surgical techniques, the results of hip arthrodesis are heavily dependent on the surgical technique chosen to perform the arthrodesis and an appropriate surgical candidate. The ideal person to consider a hip arthrodesis today includes a young patient with isolated unilateral hip arthritis ideally secondary to primary or post-traumatic degenerative arthritis. Patients should not have accompanying lumbar spine disease, ipsilateral knee pain, or contralateral hip pain. These anatomic locations have been shown in follow-up studies to have accelerated degenerative changes once the hip is fused. Young patients with a septic process or patients who have failed other hip procedures can also be considered candidates for an arthrodesis.

The importance of surgical technique on the results of hip arthrodesis must be emphasized. A successful surgical result requires not only for the hip to fuse but requires the fusion to occur in an appropriate position without violation of the abductor musculature. The optimal position of the hip following an arthrodesis is 20 to 30 degrees of hip flexion, 5 degrees of adduction, and 5 to 10 degrees of external rotation. Leg length inequality should be minimized to less than 2 cm. Depending on the patient's occupation, increased hip flexion may be considered if the patient spends a larger proportion of time in a sitting position, while less hip flexion should be considered in a patient that stands the majority of the day (manual laborer). Despite optimal hip positioning, several authors have reported low back pain and ipsilateral knee pain in greater than half the patients at long-term follow-up.

Three surgical techniques are commonly performed today for hip arthrodesis: cobra head plate, anterior plating, and dual plating. The cobra head plate, originally described by Schneider, is a technique that involves release of the abductors from the iliac crest to accommodate a cobra-shaped plate. In addition, a pelvic osteotomy is performed to improve the contact area of the femoral head on the pelvis. While fusion rates of 94% to 100% have been shown, this technique results in damage to the abductor musculature, which can be problematic should conversion to a total hip arthroplasty be attempted in the future. Anterior plating is a surgical technique that avoids damage to the hip abductor musculature and allows the fusion to occur with the patient in the supine position. Matta has reported on this technique in which an anterior Smith-Peterson approach is used and a compression plate is placed on the pelvic brim lateral to the sacroiliac joint and postero-superior iliac spine (Figure 9-2). A lag screw can also be placed from the lateral trochanteric area into the superior acetabulum and subsequently into the femoral head. Fusion rates of greater than 80% have been reported, and the results of total hip arthroplasty following this procedure are similar to a previously nonoperated hip. The dual plating technique is frequently used when patients exhibit poor bone stock, avascular bone, or are noncompliant. With the patient in a lateral position, a modified lateral approach is performed where a trochanteric osteotomy is used to elevate the abductor musculature. A lateral plate is secured to the lateral aspect of the femur and just anterior to the greater sciatic notch on the pelvis. The anterior superior iliac spine (ASIS) is then removed and a second plate is contoured and then secured distal to the ASIS and along the anterior femur before the trochanteric osteotomy is reattached.

The treatment of hip arthritis in the young patient remains challenging. In my practice, I advocate the use of hip arthrodesis in patients under the age of 25 who are employed in manual labor or in patients with recalcitrant infection in a native hip. Candidates for hip fusion must not describe pain or have radiographic evidence of arthritis in their low back, contralateral hip, or ipsilateral knee. I recommend total hip arthroplasty in young patients who are not employed in manual labor or who exhibit any of the contraindications above. I believe that hip pain in the young patient can be eliminated for several decades and that an excellent result from a total hip replacement can be expected in the future if these indications are followed and a surgical technique that does not violate the abductors is chosen.

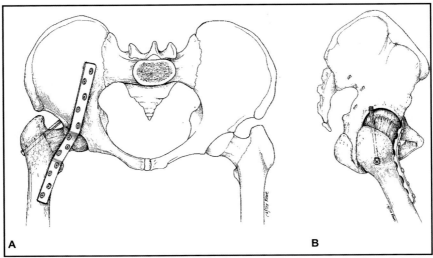

Figure 9-2. The anterior plating technique avoids damage to the abductor musculature. This procedure is performed through an anterior Smith-Peterson approach with the patient in a supine position. The supine positioning helps facilitated appropriate hip fusion positioning. (© 2002 American Academy of Orthopaedic Surgeons. Reprinted from the *Journal of the American Academy of Orthopaedic Surgeons*, Vol. 10[4], pp. 249-258 with permission.)

Bibliography

Beaule P, Matta J, Mast J. Hip arthrodesis: current indications and techniques. *JAAOS*. 2002;10(4):249-258.

Callaghan JJ, Brand RA, Pedersen DR. Hip arthrodesis: a long-term follow-up. *J Bone Joint Surg Am*. 1985;67:1328–1335.

Matta JM. Hip joint arthrodesis utilizing anterior compression plate fixation. *J Arthroplasty*. 1994;9(6):665.

Schneider R. Hip arthrodesis with the cobra head plate and pelvic osteotomy. *Reconstr Surg Traumatol*. 1974;14(0):1-37.

SECTION II

PREOPERATIVE ACETABULUM QUESTIONS

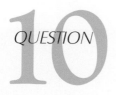
I HAVE A 34-YEAR-OLD FEMALE WITH PAIN IN HER HIP AND GROIN. HER X-RAYS AND MRI ARE "UNREMARKABLE." IS HER PAIN FROM HER HIP, AND HOW DO I KNOW?

Michael J. Taunton, MD
Robert T. Trousdale, MD

Patients with hip impingement will often have hip pain, usually exacerbated by activities or sitting. Snapping, locking, clicking, and giving away are common symptoms of labral disease.

Specific provocative maneuvers for femoroacetabular impingement (FAI) include looking for pain with flexion, internal rotation, and abduction of the hip. If there is abnormal contact between the anterior-superior acetabular rim and femoral neck, pain may be elicited. Posterior impingement is also possible and may be tested by having the patient dangle his or her legs off the end of an examination table, with the affected leg externally rotated by the examiner, and the opposite limb held flexed by the patient. In a positive exam, the femur contacts the posterior acetabular rim, eliciting pain.

Cam-type FAI occurs when a femur with an abnormal head-neck junction with insufficient head-neck offset is jammed into the acetabulum, causing shear forces on the acetabular rim and causing damage to the acetabular cartilage and labrum. This kind of impingement often occurs in patients with slipped capital femoral epiphysis (SCFE), offset abnormalities, and Perthes' disease. Many patients are males who are physically active or heavy laborers.

Pincer-type impingement is due to linear contact between the acetabular rim and labrum and the femoral head-neck junction. The labrum often ossifies, further worsening the situation by effectively deepening the acetabulum and decreasing the effective range of motion. This type is often seen in patients with coxa profunda, protrusio, and acetabular retroversion. Many of these patients are females engaging in activities that require extreme ranges of motion.

Figure 10-1. (A) The technique for obtaining the false profile view. (B) The image that is obtained.

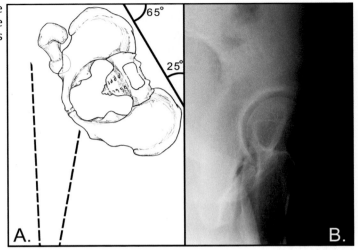

Standard anterior-posterior pelvic, frog-leg lateral, and cross-table lateral radiographs should be obtained. In certain situations a false-profile radiograph (Figure 10-1) can assess anterior femoral head coverage. The anterior posterior (AP) pelvis x-ray should be well centered and show a clear outline of the acetabulum. The coccyx should point toward the symphysis pubis, and there should be about 1 to 2 cm between them. The sourcil, the anterior and posterior walls, the teardrop, and the lateral edge of the acetabulum should be noted. Measurements may be taken to evaluate for hip dysplasia including the Tönnis angle (abnormal <10 degrees), the lateral center-edge angle of Wiberg (abnormal <25 degrees), and the anterior center-edge angle of Lequesne (abnormal <25 degrees) as measured on a false-profile radiograph. The neck shaft angle of the proximal femur is considered normal between 120 and 140 degrees.

Coxa profunda is present when the floor of the acetabular fossa is medial to the ilioischial line; protrusio is present when the medial-most femoral head overlaps the ilioischial line. The crossover sign is a sensitive and specific indicator of native acetabular retroversion. On an AP pelvis radiograph, the outlines of the edges of the anterior and posterior walls of the acetabulum should meet superiorly and laterally. In cases of acetabular retroversion, this crossover of the anterior and posterior acetabular wall outlines is more distal. Changes in the acetabular rim may also be noted. A "double line" is seen in labral ossification. An os acetabuli may also be an indicator of pathology.

Alterations of the proximal femoral anatomy, such as head-neck offset and bump formation, can be observed in addition to acetabular and labral pathology. A pistol grip deformity of the femoral head is often seen in cam-type impingement. In this situation, the superior-lateral head-neck junction is convex instead of concave. A high fovea can also indicate asphericity of the femoral head that is not able to be appreciated on the AP films. A cross-table lateral may show an abnormality in the anterior head-neck junction in cases of impingement. The alpha angle (Figure 10-2), drawn on the radial MR image, is formed by a line drawn from the center of the femoral head through the center of the femoral neck, and a line from the center of the femoral head to the femoral head-neck junction, found by the point by which the femoral neck diverges from a circle drawn around the femoral head. A normal patient's alpha angle is around 42 degrees, whereas patients with offset abnormalities this angle increases.

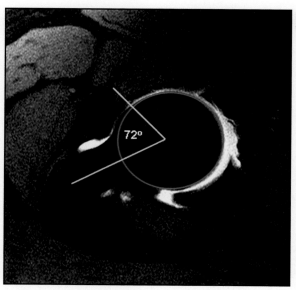

Figure 10-2. The alpha angle drawn on the radial MR image.

Computed tomography (CT) scanning allows more accurate details of the bony anatomy. If impingement or labral pathology is still suspected, contrast magnetic resonance imaging (MRI) with specialized radial sequences perpendicular to the true plane of the acetabulum is useful.

A course of nonoperative treatment for most hip pathology may be tried first. Arthroscopic assessment of the hip can include examination of both the central and peripheral compartments. The central compartment includes the labrum and all structures located further medially. Tearing of the labrum anterolaterally and damage to the acetabular cartilage is characteristic. The lesions of the labrum and any areas of chondral damage are débrided. Labral repair may be possible for specific tears. For areas of exposed subchondral bone, a microfracture technique may be performed. The peripheral compartment consists of all the structures that are lateral to the labrum but are inside the capsule. Osteophytes located around the femoral head-neck junction can be resected to restore the concavity of the femoral neck. The external portion of the labrum can also be visualized, and rim osteophytes can be resected. Some centers are altering the femoral and acetabular anatomy with the scope, but this is challenging.

Surgical dislocation of the hip has been described for treatment of FAI. The authors prefer a posterior incision (Kocher-Langenbeck). A trochanteric flip osteotomy is performed. Before subluxation or complete dislocation of the hip, an evaluation of the range of motion (ROM) should be done. This step is crucial in the decision-making process for treatment of FAI. After dislocation of the hip, the acetabular labrum and the adjacent articular cartilage are assessed, and the identified lesions are tested for partial or complete avulsions from the acetabular rim. The severity, extent, and location of these lesions should be defined, and their association with FAI should be confirmed by provocative maneuvers in flexion and internal rotation with the head relocated. The combination of anterior over coverage and the status of the labrum and the acetabular articular cartilage will determine the type of treatment of the acetabular rim. In cases of anterior over coverage contributing to FAI, as is frequent with acetabular retroversion, a resection osteoplasty of the anterosuperior rim is done. For patients presenting with FAI in the presence of acetabular retroversion, posterior wall deficiency, or at least lack of posterior over coverage, reverse periacetabular osteotomy is preferred. If the femoral head-neck junction is identified to be the cause of FAI, contouring of the femoral head and neck by excision osteoplasty is done.

Bibliography

Burnett RS, Della Rocca GJ, Prather H, Curry M, Maloney WJ, Clohisy JC. Clinical presentation of patients with tears of the acetabular labrum. *J Bone Joint Surg.* 2006;88(7):1448-1457.

Ganz R, Parvizi J, Beck M, Leunig M, Notzli H, Siebenrock KA. Femoroacetabular impingement: a cause for osteoarthritis of the hip. *Clin Orthop Relat Res.* 2003;417:112-120, 2003.

Garbuz DS, Masri BA, Haddad F, Duncan CP. Clinical and radiographic assessment of the young adult with symptomatic hip dysplasia. *Clin Orthop Relat Res.* 2004;418:18-22.

Notzli HP, Wyss TF, Stoecklin CH, Schmid MR, Treiber K, Hodler J. The contour of the femoral head-neck junction as a predictor for the risk of anterior impingement. *J Bone Joint Surg.* 2002;84(4):556-560.

Purvis SA. History and physical exam. In: Callaghan JJ, Rosenberg AG, Rubash HE, eds. *The Adult Hip.* 2nd ed. Philadelphia: Lippincott Williams & Wilkins; 2007.

Sanchez-Sotelo J, Trousdale RT, Berry DJ, Cabanela ME. Surgical treatment of DDH in adults: I non-arthroplasty options and II arthroplasty options. *JAAOS.* 2002;10(5):321-344.

Trousdale RT. Acetabular osteotomy: Indications and results. *Clin Orthopaed Rel Res.* 2004;429:182-187.

Wenger DE, Kendell KR, Miner MR, Trousdale RT. Acetabular labral tears rarely occur in the absence of bony abnormalities. *Clin Orthop Relat Res.* 2004;426:145-150.

I Have a Patient With a Loose Acetabular Component and a Moderate Amount of Bone Loss. How Can You Determine the Degree of Acetabular Bone Loss You Will Encounter Intraoperatively With Preoperative Radiographs?

Allan E. Gross, MD, FRCSC, OOnt

The classification system that I use on the acetabular side is based on loss of bone stock and leads very well into the options for each type.[1] Type I is where there is no significant loss of bone stock. This can be managed by conventional, uncemented, or even cemented components.

Type II is contained or cavitary loss of bone stock, which is a ballooning of the acetabulum, but the columns and the rim are intact. This is by far the most common type of defect and should be at least 90% of the defects seen in community practice. There are numerous options for this. All of the options may involve allograft bone, but the allograft bone can be used in a morcellized form, and the volume of graft needed can vary significantly.

* Option one would be an uncemented cup with multiple screws. The cup may have to be jumbo (over 66 mm in diameter) and should be placed into an anatomic position, which will require some use of morcellized allograft bone. The cup should have good rim support.

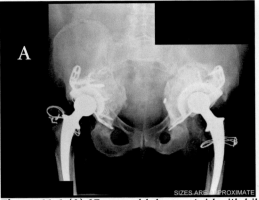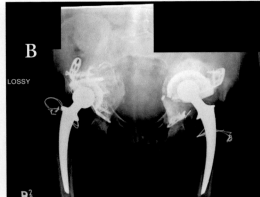

Figure 11-1. (A) 45-year-old rheumatoid with bilateral massive contained bone loss reconstructed with morcellized allograft bone protected by a cage. (B) 7 years postop, the right hip continues to do well, but the left hip has failed due to fracture of the inferior flange of the cage.

* Impaction grafting on the acetabular side is quite popular in Europe, but it has not really taken off in North America. This option uses a lot of impacted allograft bone. The impaction is firm enough that a cup can be cemented right onto the surface of the allograft bone. The champions of this technique also describe the use of wire mesh in order to make uncontained defects contained. This option is very technique dependent.

* If contact cannot be made with at least 50% bleeding host bone and a large amount of morcellized allograft bone has to be used, then consideration should be given to the use of a cage. I have published my results using a cage with massive contained bone loss, and at 5 to 7 years there is a 75% success rate[2] (Figure 11-1).

The failures are usually related to the cage and not the bone graft, and for this reason recently we have been experimenting with the use of a combination of a trabecular metal cup and the cage, the so-called cup cage construct. The object here is to create a cage that is more favorable toward bone remodeling so that permanent fixation is eventually achieved, which is not what happens with the present generation of cages. The bone graft is inserted and impacted, and then a trabecular metal cup is inserted with as many screws as is possible. If the trabecular metal cup is resting mainly on morcellized allograft bone, then it is protected by a cage that is inserted right into the trabecular metal cup. This is a relatively new technique that allows us to address these massive contained defects with this cup cage reconstruction in order to avoid the 25% failure of the cages at 5 to 7 years (Figure 11-2).

I would also like to emphasize the use of trabecular metal has allowed us to bend the rule of 50% host bone contact, and in a prospective study, our preliminary data suggest that by using trabecular metal, we can get away with less than 50% host bone contact, particularly if the host bone contact is superolaterally or in the dome of the acetabulum. The use of trabecular metal has also significantly decreased our use of roof rings.

The type III defect is uncontained or segmental, but involves less than 50% of the acetabulum. This can be addressed with 1) an oblong or a double bubble cup, 2) high hip center, 3) trabecular metal cup and augment, and 4) minor column (shelf) structural allograft with an uncemented cup. My approach today would be to use the trabecular

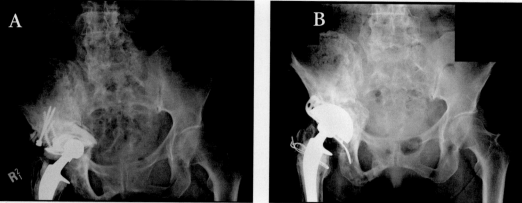

Figure 11-2. (A) Preoperative x-ray of 50-year-old male with failed reconstruction. Structural graft was still intact and made it a contained defect. (B) Reconstruction with morcellized bone, a trabecular metal cup protected by a cage.

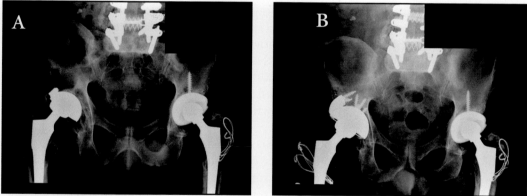

Figure 11-3. (A) Prerevision x-rays of a 15-year stable uncemented cup with an area of osteolysis superolaterally. (B) Reconstruction with a trabecular cup and a trabecular metal augment.

metal cup and augment in the elderly, low-demand patient, but I use an uncemented cup and a minor column structural allograft in the young, high-demand patient who is almost certain to come back for another revision (Figure 11-3).

The uncontained segmental defect of greater than 50% of the acetabulum is a very difficult problem to deal with, and the options are as follows: structural allograft, which has to be protected by a cage; a triflange cup, which is a custom made titanium device; and a trabecular metal cup with large trabecular metal column augments.

The type IV defect is very challenging, and the results are very guarded. The best results to date have been with the large, structural allograft protected by a cage. Once again, there is at least a 25% failure rate at 5 years, so these results are not ideal.[3] The triflanged cup, which is a custom-made titanium device, can also be used for these large defects, but the data reported have been mixed, and this device is very expensive and must be custom made. Option 3 is the use of the new trabecular metal modular system, which now has augments that resemble structural allografts and can be used both superolaterally and also anteriorly or posteriorly.

It should also be mentioned the prognosis is even more guarded if there is a type IV defect associated with a pelvic discontinuity. These pelvic discontinuities are pathological, related to osteolysis, and I doubt that they could ever be stimulated in any way to heal. My approach therefore is to span the pelvic discontinuity and hope that I can get bony ingrowth into a device that spans and splints the discontinuity. This could be done with a structural allograft if you can get it to heal at both ends, or with trabecular metal with the use of these new trabecular metal augments.

To determine preoperatively what type of defect you are dealing with, most of the time plain x-rays including an anterior posterior (AP) lateral hip and AP pelvis will suffice. Judet views are also valuable with regard to evaluating the anterior and posterior columns. These are internal and external oblique views that radiology departments should be aware of.

If you are dealing with an area of osteolysis adjacent to what appears to be a well-fixed uncemented cup, then preoperatively you should have some idea as to whether or not you are dealing with a major reconstruction, or perhaps you can leave the cup in place and do a morcellized bone grafting of the area of osteolysis, either through the screw holes in the fixed cup or by creating a window in the ilium superior to the cup. If there is any question, however, of the fixation of the cup, then I think it is better to do a complete revision. I think that you should always anticipate that the area of osteolysis is going to be larger than what you can anticipate based on your imaging studies. In this situation of osteolysis in the face of a stable cup, I think that a computed tomography (CT) scan can be particularly helpful. This will not only tell you about the size of the area of osteolysis, but it will also give you information as to whether or not the cup is well fixed and also what percent of the cup is well fixed.

It is also important to determine what part of the cup is well fixed. For example, if the area of osteolysis is mainly superolateral or in the dome, then you would want at least 50% of the cup to be well fixed in order to retain it. If it is less than that, and you try to retain the cup, it may fail shortly after the revision surgery. Another approach, particularly if you are creating a window in the ilium in order to curette the area of osteolysis, would be to use cement rather than bone graft to reconstruct the defect. The reason I say this is because using morcellized bone graft would restore bone stock for the future; however, I do not think it is reasonable to expect that biological fixation of the cup will occur through this morcellized allograft from the surrounding host bone. These defects are contained, and I think it would be more reliable to fill the defect with cement, which will adhere and provide support for the cup.

I think it is extremely important, no matter what the imaging studies may suggest, to make your final decision related to the defect and method of reconstruction at the time of surgery. I usually use a trochanteric slide for difficult acetabular reconstructions, and if there is also a difficult femoral reconstruction, then I use an extended trochanteric osteotomy, which gives me access to both the pelvic and femoral sides. A transgluteal approach can be used for the straightforward acetabular revision. A posterior approach can be used even for complex acetabular revisions because it can be easily converted to a trochanteric slide if necessary. Having approached the acetabulum, the cup and granulation tissue have to be removed, and the areas of osteolysis have to be curetted out. I then very carefully examine the medial part of the acetabulum to see whether or not there is a rim of bone protecting the pelvic contents. Next I find the ilium and trace it down anteriorly and posteriorly to evaluate the integrity of the columns and the ischium. With a trial cup placed at the correct anatomic level, which can be defined by whatever rim of the acetabulum is left and the ischium, I then decide whether my defect is contained or uncontained. If it is uncontained, I define how much of the cup is against host bone and how much of it will have to be supported by graft or augment. Then I start to do my reaming and determine once again how much bleeding host bone is available for support of the cup and where that host bone is. Then I repeat the process of using the trial cup. If the defect is completely contained but there is no reasonable host bone contact, and in order to put the cup at the right level a lot of morcellized bone is going to have to be used, then I use either the cage or the new cup cage construct. If there is a reasonable amount of host bone contact, and the trial cup appears to be stable, then a trabecular metal cup can be used. Using trabecular metal has allowed us to bend the 50% host bone contact rule down to as much as 30%, but once again it is important that contact is in an area that provides good support (ie, dome or superolateral). If the area where the cup is not supported is contained, then morcellized bone graft can be used, and if it is uncontained, then a decision has to be made as to whether or not you are going to use an augment or a minor column (shelf structural allograft).[4] If the trial cup has little or no support at the correct anatomic level, particularly related to the posterior column, then consideration has to be given either to a major column structural allograft protected by a cage or a large trabecular metal cup and the new column augments.

I would like to emphasize that it is very easy to place your cup too high or too medial unless you are absolutely sure of where you are. Take an intraoperative x-ray to confirm your position. I would also like to emphasize that in terms of your inventory of bone and implants, augments, etc, assume the worst so that you are prepared for the worst possible defect.

References

1. Saleh KJ, Holtzman J, Gafni A, et al. Development, test reliability and validation of a classification for revision hip arthroplasty. *J Ortho Res.* 2001;19(1):50–56.
2. Goodman S, Saastamoinen H, Shasha N, Gross AE. Complications of ilioischial reconstruction rings in revision total hip arthroplasty. *J Arthroplasty.* 2004;19(4):436–446.
3. Garbuz D, Morsi E, Gross AE. Revision of the acetabular component of a total hip arthroplasty with a massive structural allograft. *J Bone Joint Surg.* 1996;78A:693–697.
4. Woodgate IG, Saleh KJ, Jaroszynski G, Agnidis Z, Woodgate MM, Gross AE. Minor column structural acetabular allografts in revision hip arthroplasty. *Clin Orthop Relat Res.* 2000;371:75–85.

I Have a 72-Year-Old Patient Who Has Severe Hip Arthritis. He Had Undergone Prior Pelvic Radiation Due to Prostate Cancer. What Type of Hip Replacement Should I Perform?

Saul Magitsky, MD

The latest and most relevant study supports the use of an uncemented acetabular cup (preferably with a high scratch fit index [ie, porous tantalum or metal-foam]) with screw fixation and either a proximally coated tapered or diaphyseal engaging or cemented femoral stem. Bearing surface choices are as per surgeon's preference, postoperatively—weight bearing as tolerated (WBAT).

Radiation has deleterious effect on bone in a dose-related manner. The dosage of radiation required to cause damage to bone has been reported to be 3000 cGy for the threshold of cell change and 5000 cGy for cell death.[1] The exact mechanism, which culminates in radiation osteonecrosis, has not definitively been delineated; however, there is evidence that ionizing radiation leads to damage of the blood vessels supplying the bone and also directly affects osteoblast function and ostecyte numbers.[2] Consequent changes in the biochemical milieu of the bony environment probably lead to a decreased ability of post-irradiated bone to heal and osseointegrate.

Traditionally the options for treatment of patients with radiation necrosis include nonoperative therapy with weight-bearing restrictions, resection arthroplasty, or a total hip arthroplasty (THA). THA has been associated with a more successful outcome than the other 2 options, but the results are still not as good as a primary THA in a nonirradiated patient.

Over the years there have been several studies that have looked at patients who have undergone hip replacements after having had radiation to the pelvis. The studies have contained a high variability of components used, origin and location of malignancy, patient numbers, and gender within their groups. Because of radiation's detrimental effect on bone quality and the potential for osseointegration, it would seem natural to think that THA component fixation with cement would be a good and logical option for long-term stability. However, this has not been the case. Until recently, the results of both cemented and cementless total hip arthroplasties in these patients have been uniformly poor.[3]

Massin and Duparc[1] reported loosening of 52% acetabular and 12% femoral components in cemented hips at 69 months follow-up. Jacobs et al[4] reported a 44% (4 out of 9) failure rate of cementless acetabular components at an average of 25 months. Cho et al[2] reported 50% failure rates for acetabular components in both cementless cups (7 out of 14) and cemented roof-ring constructs (2 out of 4) at a mean of 59 months follow-up. This study additionally identified the latency period from radiation treatment to onset of hip pain as a statistically significant predictor of acetabular component failure. The authors postulated that the shorter latency period could be due to symptoms arising from a direct injury to a focal bony area, which can be adequately addressed by curettage at the time of surgery, versus a longer latency period, which may be a result of the remodeling reparative process of creeping substitution that further weakens the underlying bone in an inadequate attempt to compensate for the osteonecrosis. The bony inadequacies created by such a diffuse resorptive process would be much more difficult to fully address with curettage at the time of the procedure, increasing the possibility that repair or additional necrosis could further progress even after surgery.

More recently, however, 2 studies have reported encouraging results. Rose et al[5] described a group of 11 patients (12 hips), all of whom had therapeutic pelvic radiation (average cGy 5890) to treat an underlying malignancy at an average of 155 months prior to the procedure. All of the patients were treated with a trabecular metal acetabular revision shell with screw augmentation (average 4 screws) and a cemented liner. One stem was fully porous-coated, the rest were cemented. At a 24- to 48-month follow-up, there were no clinical failures (no progressive or complete radiolucencies, no detectable component migration). The authors acknowledge the limitations of short follow-up and a small sample size (12 hips), but nevertheless these results are certainly encouraging in the short term. Porous tantalum has a high coefficient of friction due to its structure, and once augmented with multiple screw fixation, these constructs may provide the necessary rigid fixation for early bone ingrowth.

The other report that gives hope for improved longer term results is by Kim et al.[3] This is the first study to look exclusively at a cohort consisted of 58 patients (66 hips) postirradiated patients with histologically confirmed adeno-CA of prostate who underwent uncemented hip arthroplasties. The average age of the patients was 74. Underlying diagnosis was osteonecrosis of the femoral head in 31 (47%) hips and degenerative joint disease in 35 (53%). The average dose of radiation administered was cGy 7065, and the average follow-up was 4.8 years (2 to 7.5). All patients underwent uncemented THA with plasma-sprayed cups (18 with screw supplementation) and proximally coated collarless tapered femoral stems. At the latest follow-up, all uncemented femoral and acetabular components showed evidence of osseointegration and were deemed stable. Both Harris hip scores and SF-36 summary measures for physical and mental health showed statistically significant improvements in all 51 patients. There were 3 reoperations (infection, femoral stem subsidence, and periprosthetic femur fracture after a fall), none of which were deemed to be related to irradiation.

Conclusion

Individuals with hip disease and a history of previous pelvic irradiation are a challenging subset of patients that an orthopedist is on occasion called to care for. Although previously reported results have been uniformly poor, and longer follow-ups of more recent ones are needed, the latest studies certainly give encouragement and point in a direction of treatment rationale with potentially improved clinical outcomes. The patients must be made aware of the poor clinical outcomes reported in the past and the short nature of follow-up in the more encouraging recent reports. Additionally, it is imperative to make the patient aware that if the operation fails due to infection, component loosening, or fracture of the pelvis, resection arthroplasty is probably the last and most prudent treatment option left.

References

1. Massin P, Duparc J. Total hip replacement in irradiated hips: a retrospective study of 71 cases. *J Bone Joint Surg Br.* 1995;77(6):847–852.
2. Cho MR, Kwun KW, Lee DH, Kim SY, Kim JD. Latent period best predicts acetabular cup failure after total hip arthroplasties in radiated hips. *Clin Orthop Relat Res.* 2005;438:165–170.
3. Kim KI, Klein GR, Sleeper J, Dicker AP, Rothman RH, Parvizi J. Uncemented total hip arthroplasty in patients with a history of pelvic irradiation for prostate cancer. *J Bone Joint Surg Am.* 2007;89(4):798–805.
4. Jacobs JJ, Kull LR, Frey GA, et al. Early failure of acetabular components inserted without cement after previous pelvic irradiation. *J Bone Joint Surg Am.* 1995;77(12):1829–1835.
5. Rose PS, Halasy M, Trousdale RT, et al. Preliminary results of tantalum acetabular components for THA after pelvic radiation. *Clin Orthop Relat Res.* 2006;453:195–198.

I Have a Patient With Start-Up Groin Pain 5 Years After Surgery, and I Think the Acetabular Component Is Loose. How Can I Tell for Sure?

Amanda D. Marshall, MD

Clinical suspicion of acetabular loosening is heightened with the above-described symptoms of start-up groin pain. A clinical exam is helpful in ruling out other groin pain generators such as the possibility of a lumbar etiology or iliopsoas tendon irritation. However, in a symptomatic patient, clinical test sensitivities for diagnosing loosening are too low to replace a radiological evaluation as the "gold standard."[1] Therefore, your next step after the clinical exam is a detailed radiographic analysis consisting of the standard antero-posterior (AP) pelvis, AP and lateral hip views. Paramount is the ability to compare the current x-ray with an older film taken closer to the time of surgery. Although there is no test with 100% accuracy, radiographic comparison is the most "sure" way to determine if the acetabular component is loose.

The traditional radiological method of determining the stability of the cup is based on a zonal analysis originally described by DeLee and Charnley.[2] They recognized the problem of "radiologic demarcation" at the cemented bone interface of cemented Charnley cups as early as 1962. This was described as a dark line between the radiopaque cement and the bone of the acetabulum. In their analysis of 141 hips, the authors determined both the width of this radiolucency as well as the distribution around the circumference of the socket. On an anterior posterior (AP) radiograph of the pelvis, this distribution was categorized into 3 zones (Figure 13-1): I (superior/lateral), II (central), and III (inferior/medial). For an average follow-up of 10 years, 69.5% demonstrated radiolucencies and 9.2% showed migration. Noted was an association of increased probability of loosening with a greater distribution of radiolucencies. Since this early article, other authors have helped establish the criteria of an impending failure of the cemented acetabular component. In 1983, Dorr et al defined it as a continuous radiolucent line at least 2 mm in width

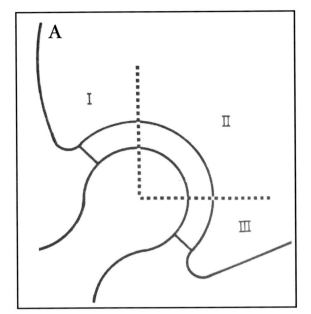

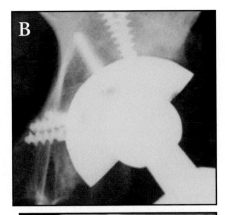

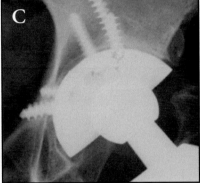

Figure 13-1. (A) Radiographic acetabular zones. (Adapted from DeLee JG, Charnley J. Radiological demarcation of cemented sockets in total hip replacement. *Clin Orthop Relat Res.* 1976;121:20–32.) (B and C) Progression of a radiolucent line seen over a 2-year period.

along all 3 zones of the circumference of the bone-cement interface.[3] Hodgkinson et al further characterized this relationship between radiolucencies and loosening by demonstrating that a gap >1 mm involving the lateral two thirds of the cup was predictive of failure.[4] Another indicator of a loose cup is migration, whether it is superior or medial. Migration <3 mm, however, is within the limits of error for measurement and radiographic technique. Therefore, limits in the literature have generally been 4 mm. Other variables to look for when determining cup stability are cement fractures, cup breakage, or progressive tilt of the cup. I caution you on putting too great an emphasis on changes in tilt. Two degrees is a commonly accepted margin of error, but small technique changes in the caudad-cephalad plane between subsequent films can also result in perceived tilt progression. Prior films are most helpful in documenting progression of these variables. In summary, when assessing cemented acetabular components, my criteria for suspected loosening are any of the following:

* A continuous radiolucency ≥1 mm in zones I, II, and III.
* A radiolucent line >1 mm in zones I and II.
* Migration ≥4 mm superiorly or medially.
* Cement fractures.

When assessing cementless acetabular components, the same basic principles of radiographic assessment apply. The 2 predictors of loosening are progressive radiolucencies and migration. One factor that needs to be mentioned in cementless cup assessment is the difference between gaps and radiolucent lines. A gap is defined as an area at which the cup was not in direct contact with the bone seen on the immediate postoperative films. A radiolucent line is defined as a space that develops on subsequent radiographs in zones where no gap had previously existed or after gaps had resolved. The association between gaps and subsequent presence of radiolucent lines has not been consistently demonstrated in the literature. Another factor to consider is the more subtle radiolucent lines when associated with progression of polyethylene wear. Studies have demonstrated that the main predictors of loosening[5] for uncemented acetabular components are as follows:

* Radiolucencies that progressed or initially appeared after 2 years.
* A continuous radiolucent line in zones I to III.
* A radiolucent line >2 mm in any one zone.
* Migration (linear change >3 mm or rotational change >8 degrees).

In an effort to better assess the osseointegration of porous-coated uncemented cups, a recent study by Moore et al[6] introduces a 5-sign system as another radiographic tool. Their 5 criteria are 1) absence of radiolucent lines, 2) presence of a superolateral buttress, 3) an inferomedial buttress, 4) medial stress shielding, and 5) radial trabeculae. The authors reviewed 119 total hip arthroplasties undergoing revision surgery and correlated the intraoperative findings to those of the post-primary and pre-revision radiographs. These signs were reliable predictors of bony ingrowth, especially when used in combination. The positive predictive value was 97% when 3 of the 5 signs were present. This system is relatively new and is not yet universally accepted. However, I feel this approach to assessing bony ingrowth has a sound scientific basis of adaptive changes of the bony acetabulum in response to loads applied via a well-integrated cup. Similarly to Engh's criteria to assess porous-coated femoral stems, additional studies will likely add more validity to this system, translating into a commonly used radiographic assessment tool.[7]

Overall, the diagnosis of a loose acetabular component is based on a combination of clinical suspicion, physical exam findings, and radiographs. However, occasionally there is still some uncertainty as to whether or not the acetabular component is the etiology of the pain. In this circumstance, additional tests are available. These include bone scans, digital subtraction arthrography, and positron emission tomography (PET). Of these, bone scans are the most readily available in my institution and therefore, I have used them as supplemental indicators of suspected loosening. The literature reports a very wide range of diagnostic accuracy. It is a highly sensitive test (64% to 100%) but not very specific (60% to 80%), as increased uptake is seen in various conditions including infection, heterotopic bone formation, stress fracture, modulus mismatch, reflex sympathetic dystrophy, tumor, and metabolic bone disease. If the bone scan is normal (which is rare), loosening of the cup is very unlikely. A more recent diagnostic test used primarily in the larger academic institutions has been PET scanning. In addition to detecting loosening, it has also shown some promising potential in differentiating between aseptic loosening and infection.

Conclusion

Clinical examination and plain radiographs are still the mainstay in the diagnosis of a loose acetabular component.

References

1. Roder C, Eggli S, Aebi M, Busato A. The validity of clinical examination in the diagnosis of loosening of components in total hip arthroplasty. *J Bone Joint Surg.* 2003;85-B:37–44.
2. DeLee JG, Charnley J. Radiological demarcation of cemented sockets in total hip replacement. *Clin Orthop Relat Res.* 1976;121:20–32.
3. Dorr LD, Takei GK, Conaty JP. Total hip arthroplasties in patients less than forty-five years old. *J Bone Joint Surg.* 1983;65-A:474–479.
4. Hodgkinson JP, Shelley P, Wrobleski BM. The correlation between the roentgenographic appearance and operative findings at the bone-cement junction of the socket in Charnley low friction arthroplasties. *Clin Orthop Relat Res.* 1988;228:105–109.
5. Udomkiat P, Wan Z, Dorr LD. Comparison of preoperative radiographs and intraoperative findings of fixation of hemispheric porous-coated sockets. *J Bone Joint Surg.* 2001;83-A:1865–1870.
6. Moore MS, McAuley JP, Young AM, Engh CA. Radiographic signs of osseointegration in porous-coated acetabular components. *Clin Orthop Relat Res.* 2006;444:176–183.
7. Engh CA, Bobyn JD, Glassman AH. Porous-coated hip replacement: the factors governing bone ingrowth, stress shielding, and clinical results. *JBJS.* 1987;69B:45-55.

I HAVE A PATIENT WITH A CROWE TYPE III HIP DYSPLASIA. WHERE DO I PLACE THE ACETABULAR COMPONENT?

Duncan Jacks, MD
Alexander Siegmeth, MD, FRCS
Bassam A. Masri, MD, FRCSC

Total hip arthroplasty in the setting of developmental dysplasia of the hip can be technically demanding with the need for complex reconstruction of the acetabular deficiency. A thorough understanding of the bony deficiency is required to assist in preoperative planning and to minimize complications.

Crowe et al classified developmental dysplasia of the hip based on the degree of femoral head migration in relationship to the true acetabulum. Type I hips have less than 50% subluxation, Type II have between 50% and 75% subluxation, Type III have between 75% and 100% subluxation, and Type IV have complete dislocation. The Crowe Type III dysplastic hip presents a specific challenge due to severe bony deficiency in the superolateral acetabulum. Controversy exists over the optimal placement of the acetabular component.

One option is to place a small porous cup in a superior position ("high hip center") where it may be possible to obtain better lateral bone coverage and minimize excessive soft tissue tension. However, unacceptably high loosening rates have been noted; therefore, if at all possible, we prefer to restore the hip center to its anatomic position ("true acetabulum"). This medial and inferior location diminishes joint reaction forces, facilitates limb lengthening, and in most cases utilizes the best available bone stock.

From a technical standpoint, once the hip is dislocated you may have difficulty visualizing the true acetabulum. A ledge of bone often separates the true acetabulum from the false one and can help guide further inferior dissection. The lower edge of the teardrop and the transverse acetabular ligament must be located by inserting a blunt inferior retractor. This can help ensure that dissection is inferior enough to place the component in the true acetabulum. The depth of the acetabulum can also be difficult to appreciate. It is important to remove the pulvinar to expose the cotyloid fossa in order to assess the depth of the medial wall and to safely ream the acetabulum. One trick to identify the thickness of bone in the true acetabulum is to drill with a small drill bit and then measure the thickness of the medial wall with a depth gauge. This prevents excessive bone removal from the medial wall. For most cases, the component needs to be medialized as much as possible, even if a minimal amount of the medial wall is breached. We would not recommend deliberate excessive reaming of the medial wall. If there is a small breach, this should be grafted.

The dysplastic acetabulum can be quite shallow, and very small acetabular components may be required. We usually start with a very small reamer and then progressively ream up to enlarge the acetabulum, with the anteroposterior dimension of the true acetabulum determining that size of the final component. By necessity, due to the dysplastic nature of the socket, once reaming is completed, there will be a superolateral bony deficiency that may need to be addressed. It is not important to achieve 100% bony coverage of the acetabulum, particularly superolaterally. What is important, however, is to have enough support superolaterally that the acetabular component is stable. Once a good press-fit is achieved, the socket has to be able to resist moderate stress applied against the superior rim. If the component is unstable and tends to tip into abduction with mild to moderate pressure on the superior rim, bone stock superolaterally should be augmented. For the most part, if there is less than 20% to 30% of uncoverage, the socket will be stable. When a large superolateral defect remains, our preference is to use bulk femoral autograft with careful graft preparation to ensure congruity. We aim to fix the graft using cortical screws beneath a solid buttress of host bone. Partial support is usually provided by the superior lip of the false acetabulum. We then shape the graft and host acetabulum using hemispherical reamers, with caution to not excessively torque the graft. If a significant proportion (>50%) of the socket needs to be covered with allograft, then consideration should be given to using cement, as bony ingrowth into the dead bone graft is unlikely. Alternatively, while not in common use for this indication, trabecular metal implants and a trabecular metal augment may be used instead of bone to achieve support. So-called double-bubble cups have been used with variable results. We prefer to not use them, as they are unpredictable.

Acetabular reconstruction in the Crowe III dysplastic hips can be challenging. When possible, We attempt to place a small, uncemented acetabular component in the true acetabulum. Augmentation with bulk allograft or a trabecular metal augment should be considered when more than 30% of the cup is uncovered. Other options such as the cotyloplasty technique and the high hip center have been used but are not universally accepted.

Bibliography

Crowe JF, Mani VJ, Ranawat CS. Total hip replacement in congenital dislocation and dysplasia of the hip. *J Bone Joint Surg.* 1979;61A:15-23.

Haddad FS, Masri BA, Garbuz DS, Duncan CP. Primary total hip replacement of the dysplastic hip. *J Bone Joint Surg.* 1999;81A:1462-1482.

Kobayashi S, Saito N, Nawata M, Horiuchi H, Iorio R, Takaoka K. Total hip arthroplasty with bulk femoral head autograft for acetabular reconstruction in DDH. *J Bone Joint Surg.* 2004;86 A Suppl 1:11-17.

Pagnano MW, Hanssen AD, Lewallen DG, Shaughnessy WJ. The effect of superior placement of the acetabular component on the rate of loosening after total hip arthroplasty. *J Bone Joint Surg.* 1996;78A:1004-1014.

Stans A, Pagnano M, Shaughnessy W, Hanssen A. Results of total hip arthroplasty for Crowe Type III developmental hip dysplasia. *Clin Orthop Relat Res.* 1998;348:149-157.

I Have a Patient With a Pelvic Discontinuity. What Can I Expect to Find Intraoperatively, and How Should I Plan on Reconstructing This Defect?

Scott M. Sporer, MD

A pelvic discontinuity occurs when the superior hemipelvis is disconnected from the inferior hemipelvis (Figure 15-1). This distinct bone defect must be identified at the time of revision surgery and treated appropriately in order to obtain implant stability and to optimize patient outcomes. Pelvic discontinuity occurs most commonly either preoperatively due to severe bone loss from osteolysis or intraoperatively following component insertion. Risk factors for pelvic discontinuity include female patients, patients with rheumatoid arthritis, and patients with prior radiation. Radiographic signs of a pelvic discontinuity include a visible fracture line through the anterior and posterior columns, medial translation of the inferior hemipelvis relative to the superior hemipelvis, and asymmetry of the obturator foramen on an anterior posterior radiograph secondary to inferior hemipelvis rotation. I always perform an intraoperative assessment for a pelvic discontinuity during an acetabular revision by placing a Cobb elevator along the posterior column and applying a posteriorly directed force. A transverse fracture line is most frequently observed in a discontinuity and can be seen as motion between the 2 hemipelvis.

Berry et al have classified pelvic discontinuity into 3 categories: Type IVa is associated with cavitary bone loss or mild segmental bone loss, Type IVb is associated with segmental bone loss, and Type IVc is associated with previous pelvic irradiation. Plating of the posterior column along with a porous hemispherical component was recommended for Type IVa defects while particulate bone graft or a bulk structural allograft supported with an antiprotrusio cage was recommended for most Type IVb and IVc defects. I believe

Figure 15-1. A pelvic discontinuity occurs when the superior and inferior hemipelvis are not connected. This occurs most frequently due to bone loss from osteolysis or secondary to fracture during component insertion.

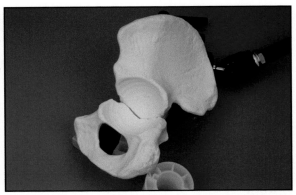

that the treatment of a pelvic discontinuity should be dependent not only upon the amount of host bone loss but also whether or not adequate biological potential exists to unite the superior and inferior hemipelvis. The 4 most common types of pelvic dissociation that I encounter are 1) acute, which occurs during component insertion; 2) chronic with minimal bone loss; 3) chronic with moderate/severe bone loss; and 4) discontinuity secondary to pathologic bone (radiation/tumor). There is generally minimal bone loss when an acute intraoperative fracture occurs. In this situation, I recommend the use of a posterior column plate to provide compression at the site of the discontinuity and direct bone apposition. Once the discontinuity has been stabilized, a hemispherical component can be inserted and multiple screws placed into the superior and inferior hemipelvis. I prefer to use an acetabular component that requires the use of cement to secure the liner since the cement will adhere to the screws and result in a "locked" screw (Figure 15-2). I prefer to treat a chronic discontinuity with minimal bone loss with a similar technique. However, I make sure that prior to acetabular preparation, all fibrous tissue from the discontinuity has been removed and that particulate bone graft has been placed. A chronic discontinuity with moderate/severe bone loss is more difficult to treat since direct bone contact between the superior and inferior hemipelvis is unlikely. As a result, it is unlikely that bone union across the discontinuity will occur. I believe that there are 2 options to manage this difficult situation. A posterior column plate can be used to stabilize the pelvis before either bulk allograft or particulate allograft is inserted and subsequently supported by a cage (Figure 15-3). I have abandoned this technique except in the most extreme cases of bone loss due to late cage failure. An alternative option is to use a highly porous acetabular component and to distract the superior and inferior hemipelvis across the discontinuity. This technique does not allow healing of the discontinuity, but rather relies upon the inherent strength of the acetabular component. In order for this technique to be successful, micromotion must be minimized until bone from both the superior and inferior hemipelvis has had time to grow into the component.

Pelvic discontinuity in association with radiation remains a difficult problem to treat due to the poor biologic healing potential. In this situation, I prefer to use the "cup-cage" technique described by Gross et al. In this situation, the discontinuity is stabilized and a highly porous-coated cup is placed into the irradiated acetabulum. A cage is then placed over the cup to provide immediate mechanical stability while a polyethylene liner is cemented into the cage.

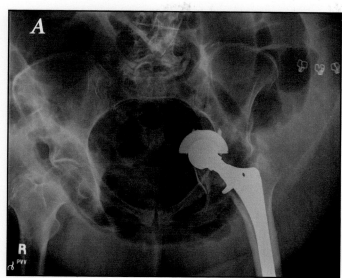

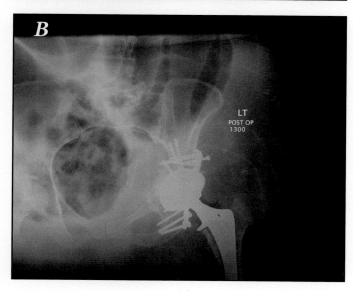

Figure 15-2. A 73-year-old female who underwent a primary total hip arthroplasty. (A) Postoperative radiograph demonstrating medial component migration with an associated pelvic discontinuity. (B) Adequate bone remained to place a posterior column plate and obtain direct bone contact prior to placing a hemispherical acetabular component.

Figure 15-3. A 56-year-old female who underwent an acetabular revision. (A) Postoperative radiograph demonstrating severe segmental bone loss and associated pelvic discontinuity. (B) A bulk allograft was used to span the defect while a cage was used to protect the allograft until bone union occurred.

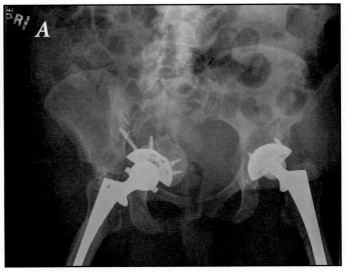

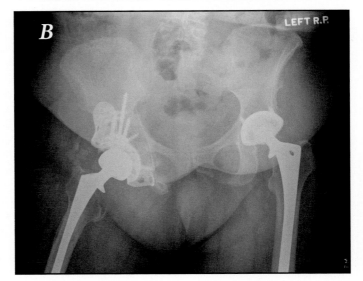

Bibliography

Berry DJ, Lewallen DG, Hanssen AD, Cabanela ME. Pelvic discontinuity in revision total hip arthroplasty. *J Bone Joint Surg Am.* 1999;81(12):1692-1702.

Gross AE, Goodman SB. Rebuilding the skeleton: the intraoperative use of trabecular metal in revision total hip arthroplasty. *J Arthroplasty.* 2005;20(4 Suppl 2):91-93.

I Have a Patient Who Is 10 Years Postoperative From a Hip Replacement With Severe Polyethylene Wear and Retroacetabular Osteolysis. When Do I Intervene With a Polyethylene Liner Exchange?

Raju S. Ghate, MD

Osteolysis continues to plague the long-term survival of total hip arthroplasty (THA). All common bearing surfaces have been found to have the ability to cause osteolysis. While initially thought of as cement disease, we now know osteolysis to be a macrophage-mediated response to wear debris, classically polyethylene.[1-3]

Published data suggest that patients with greater than 0.1 mm/year of polyethylene wear have an increased risk of developing osteolysis.[4] However, not all patients with significant polyethylene wear have significant osteolysis. The reasons for this at this time are not completely understood. When osteolysis does occur, quantifying the amount of retroacetabular lysis can be difficult at best with plain radiographs alone. Puri et al have shown computed tomography (CT) with metal artifact minimization to be more sensitive and accurate than plain radiographs alone.[5] It also allows for better preoperative planning in terms of understanding the extent and location of osteolysis. Beyond that, CT can also be used as a tool to monitor progression. Further work has demonstrated that these lesions tend to progress at a rate of approximately 12% per year.

Patients with polyethylene wear and associated osteolysis can be difficult to indicate for surgical intervention, as the patients are rarely symptomatic until catastrophic failure occurs such as periprosthetic fracture or loosening of the acetabular component.[6] It is for that reason a CT scan along with serial radiographs demonstrating progression are help-ful in counseling the patient as well as comforting the surgeon that operative intervention is warranted.

The ideal time to intervene is a well-fixed cup with a functional locking mechanism, demonstrated progressive wear with or without significant osteolysis, in a well-posi-tioned cup that is of course modular. Data and logic strongly support that isolated liner exchange is much easier and has better outcomes than complete acetabular revision.[7]

Treatment of the osteolytic lesions is controversial. Most surgeons would agree that curettage is a minimum, and grafting while optional is preferred. Recent work by Puri et al has demonstrated a reduction in size of the osteolytic lesions on CT at 2 years after liner change and grafting with a variety of graft options.[8] Reconstitution of retroacetabu-lar bone stock can be important should future revision be required. Our grafting method uses cancellous chips placed through screw holes with or without demineralized bone matrix (DBX) for large lesions and DBX alone for small lesions.

Difficulty arises when a damaged or poor locking mechanism is present in a well-fixed, well-positioned cup. However, there are data to support the use of cement to secure the cup. Haft et al have demonstrated that a 2-mm cement mantle with burring of the backside of the polyethylene and in some cases the inside of the metal shell to allow for cement integration is as strong or stronger than most locking mechanisms.[9]

Further difficulty exists when a nonmodular or monoblock acetabular component has significant polyethylene wear and osteolysis. In that setting with a well-fixed cup, ream-ers can be used to remove the remaining polyethylene, and a new liner can be cemented into the well-fixed shell.

Conclusion

Our current algorithm for management of severe polyethylene wear and osteolysis is a CT to understand the size and location of the lesions followed by liner change and graft-ing when the cup is well positioned and stable. If the locking mechanism is disrupted, we recommend cementing into an otherwise well-fixed shell.

References

1. Archibeck MJ, Jacobs JJ, Rocbuck KA, Glant TT. The basic science of periprosthetic osteolysis. *Instr Course Lect.* 2001;50:185-195.
2. Bankston AB, Cates H, Ritter MA, Keating EM, Faris PM. Polyethylene wear in total hip arthroplasty. *Clin Orthop.* 1995;317:7-13.
3. Charnley J, Halley DK. Rate of wear in total hip replacement. *Clin Orthop Relat Res.* 1975;112:170-179.
4. Dumbleton JH, Manley MT, Edidin AA. A literature review of the association between wear rate and osteolysis in total hip arthroplasty. *J Arthroplasty.* 2002;17(5):649-661.
5. Puri L, Wixson RL, Stern SH, Kohli J, Hendrix RW, Stulberg SD. Use of helical computed tomography for the assessment of acetabular osteolysis after total hip arthroplasty. *J Bone Joint Surg Am.* 2002;84-A(4):609-614.
6. Lavernia CJ. Cost-effectiveness of early surgical intervention in silent osteolysis. *J Arthroplasty.* 1998;13(3):277-279.
7. Schmalzried TP, Fowble VA, Amstutz HC. The fate of pelvic osteolysis after reoperation: no recurrence with lesional treatment. *Clin Orthop Relat Res.* 1998;350:128-137.

8. Puri L, Lapinski B, Wixson RL, Lynch J, Hendrix R, Stulberg SD. Computed tomographic follow-up evaluation of operative intervention for periacetabular lysis. *J Arthroplasty.* 2006;21(6 Suppl 2):78-82.
9. Haft GF, Heiner AD, Dorr LD, Brown TD, Callaghan JJ. A biomechanical analysis of polyethylene liner cementation into a fixed metal acetabular shell. *J Bone Joint Surg Am.* 2003;85-A(6):1100-1110.

I Have a Patient Who Is 10 Years Postoperative From a Loose Acetabular Component. When Do I Need to Use More Than a Hemispherical Component?

Brian P. Murphy, MD, MS

When planning an acetabular revision, preoperative planning is essential. The first step is to definitively determine what components are in place and to have the appropriate replacements available. If planning on leaving the femoral stem, having the correct femoral head sizes, lengths, and tapers is important. The next step is to make sure that you have good quality plain films. An anterior posterior (AP) pelvis, AP, and frog leg lateral of the hip and shoot through lateral are often times sufficient. Judet films can sometimes help better delineate the status of the anterior and posterior columns. Occasionally, computed tomography (CT) scans with techniques to reduce metal artifact can assist in determining the amount and location of bone loss. Ultimately, intraoperative assessment will determine the type of reconstruction needed.

I have found the Paprosky classification very useful in determining preoperatively the likelihood of needing to augment a hemispherical cup.[1] The 4 radiographic landmarks that are used as key indicators to the location and extent of bone loss are the acetabular teardrop, Kohler's line, the presence or absence of ischial lysis, and vertical migration of the socket. The teardrop represents the inferior portion of the anterior column and medial wall. Kohler's line represents the medial wall and superior portion of the anterior column. Ischial lysis, best seen on the shoot through lateral, suggests compromise of the posterior column. Vertical migration of more than 3 cm reflects damage to the superior dome of the acetabulum and possibly a portion of the superior posterior column depending on the direction of migration. When evaluating these landmarks, you are trying to determine if there is sufficient support around the rim of the acetabulum and adequate viable host-bone area to create an environment suitable for cementless fixation of a hemispherical cup. Rim support is needed to securely and rigidly hold the cup long enough for bony ingrowth. You need 2 points separated by enough distance (ie, posterior/superior to anterior/inferior) to allow a press-fit. If that can be achieved, the next question is whether or not the necessary 50% host-bone contact is present to provide enough surface area for long-term biologic fixation.[2] If it is not present, a hemispherical cup will not work, and more advanced reconstruction techniques may be necessary.

Intraoperatively, the first step is to remove the component with as little damage to host bone as possible. The next step is aggressive debridement of membranous and fibrous tissue as well as osteolytic bone. Once this has been accomplished, a reamer should be placed in the desired final cup position. Often, anatomic landmarks are distorted or missing, making this difficult. Locating the obturator foramen can help determine cup height. Accurate patient positioning prior to the start of the case will help to determine the correct anteversion and abduction. Although tempting, it is important to avoid placing the cup in a position of maximal coverage at the expense of orientation. Begin reaming, preferentially maintaining the posterior column even if at the expense of the anterior column. As you increase reamer size to achieve quality contact in one dimension (top to bottom), you must pay close attention to what you are losing in another (front to back). Once it appears that you will no longer increase bony contact or support with increased reamer size, it is time to trial. Attempt to impact a trial into the desired location. If it is stable enough to allow a trial reduction and it remains in good anatomic position, you are finished. A hemispherical cup is sufficient. However, if the trial is not supported enough for rigid stability, augmentation is needed.

The choice for augmentation of a hemispherical cup has traditionally been structural allograft. Recently, tantalum augments have become available, which may provide a feasible alternative. The advantages of allograft are availability and restoration of bone stock for possible future revisions. The disadvantages are potential resorption leading to an unsupported cup and disease transmission. Dewal et al[3] found that the keys to successful use of structural allograft were adequate host-bone contact, component screws with good host-bone purchase, and the alignment of graft trabeculae with those of the host ilium. They had no revisions and graft incorporation at an average follow-up of 6.8 years. These data illustrate that structural allograft is a good option.

Trabecular metal augments have advantages as well. The material has a greater surface roughness increasing the intraoperative scratch fit, and the biocompatibility of tantalum appears to create an excellent environment for ingrowth. The augments are available in different shapes and sizes that can be shaped and positioned for maximum host-bone contact, secured with screws into host bone, and then cemented to the hemispherical cup. If the augments ingrow and are securely attached to the cup, it is no different than if the cup had ingrown itself. A disadvantage is that there are currently no mid- or long-term studies to support these purported advantages.

Conclusion

The importance of determining what implants are in place and having the correct components available for exchange or replacement cannot be underestimated. Equally important is the meticulous preoperative examination of x-rays to help tentatively determine if a hemispherical cup will suffice. However, be prepared to find more bone loss than expected, and have the necessary equipment and components available to handle it. With proper preparation and planning, challenging acetabular revisions can be managed.

References

1. Paprosky WG, Perona PG, Lawrence JM. Acetabular defect classification and surgical reconstruction in revision arthroplasty: a 6-year follow-up evaluation. *J Arthroplasty*. 1994;9(1):33–44.
2. Della Valle CJ, Berger RA, Rosenberg AG, Galante JO. Cementless acetabular reconstruction in revision total hip arthroplasty. *Clin Orthop*. 2004;420:96–100.
3. Dewal H, Chen F, Su E, Di Cesare PE. Use of structural bone graft with cementless acetabular cups in total hip arthroplasty. *J Arthroplasty*. 2003;18(1):23–28.

SECTION III

PREOPERATIVE
FEMUR QUESTIONS

I Have a Patient With a Crowe Type IV Hip Dysplasia. What Femoral Component Do I Use and When Do I Need to Do a Femoral Shortening Osteotomy?

James Slover, MD, MS

In the Crowe classification of hip dysplasia,[1] Crowe IV hips represent the most severely affected hips with complete dislocation of the femoral head from the acetabulum and with vertical displacement of the femur of a distance greater than 100% of the diameter of the femoral head from the inter-teardrop line. Due to the abnormal biomechanical forces on the dislocated and vertically displaced Crowe IV femur, it often demonstrates excessive anteversion, a narrowed or angulated femoral canal, an increased valgus femoral neck angle, and a posteriorly displaced greater trochanter, making femoral reconstruction more challenging than for a typical primary osteoarthritic hip.[2]

Careful preoperative templating and planning is necessary to ensure the success of this operation. Typically either uncemented fully porous-coated stems, fluted stems with porous-coated proximal sleeves, or cemented stems are used. Nonmodular implants may be difficult to implant with appropriate correction of anteversion due to restriction of rotation of the implant in the metaphyseal region. Consequently, I generally prefer modular stems with a porous-coated proximal sleeve and a fluted stem in this situation, provided adequate fixation of the proximal sleeve can be achieved. This allows for easy correction of femoral anteversion and for preparation of the proximal femur and proximal sleeve implantation before making the osteotomy, as the osteotomy site will be below the distal-most level of the proximal sleeve. Preparation is easier with the femur intact, and this should be completed prior to making the osteotomy. If this type of implant is used, you must be sure distal fixation is adequately achieved by a tight fit, which is evident by closure of the clothespin tip. Intraoperative x-rays should definitely be used to ensure adequate fill of the canal in this situation.

In order to restore the normal biomechanical forces on the reconstructed acetabulum and bone stock considerations, it is often desirable to restore the hip center to its normal location. The surrounding soft tissues, including the hip musculature, and nervous structures can often be significantly contracted. Overlengthening of these structures can produce significant leg length discrepancies, overtighten the musculature making it difficult or impossible to reduce the femoral head, or damage the femoral or sciatic nerve, which is capable of stretching finite amounts. There have been reports in the literature of sciatic nerve injuries with lengthening of 2 to 4 cm.[3] If reconstruction will require lengthening of greater than 4 cm, a femoral shortening osteotomy should be completed. It may be required for smaller lengthenings as well. Surgeons planning a total hip replacement for patients with Crowe IV hip dysplasia should be prepared to do a femoral shortening osteotomy, even if the required lengthening is less than 4 cm, in the event that the contracted soft tissues will not allow reduction of the reconstructed femur or the tension of the sciatic nerve is deemed to be too great, risking nerve injury. Surgical approach is a matter of surgeon preference, although a posterior approach allows for easier assessment of sciatic nerve tension.

Cemented fixation should be used with great care in this situation to ensure no interposition of cement in the osteotomy site, which will prevent healing. Concerns for this complication make the use of modular uncemented implants even more preferred after subtrochanteric osteotomy. I prefer modular implants with proximal sleeve fixation to nonmodular fully porous-coated stems because it is often easier to achieve customized fixation with these implants, rather than relying on diaphyseal fixation with fully porous-coated stems, given the femoral deformities previously discussed. There are 2 primary options for femoral shortening osteotomy. A greater trochanteric osteotomy can be performed in combination with proximal femoral shortening. This can be done sequentially if necessary. In this case, the femoral component is implanted in the distal femur, and the greater trochanter is reapproximated by the same techniques used for standard trochanteric osteotomies. This has the advantage of comfort for most arthroplasty surgeons. The disadvantage is that it requires the removal of metaphyseal bone, leaving the cortical diaphysis as the only remaining area of fixation for the femoral component, which often requires the use of a cemented or fully porous-coated stem, making future reconstruction, which is often necessary in young patients, more difficult. In addition, there is a risk of nonunion of the greater trochanter to the diaphyseal femur, which can be very problematic for the patient.

A second, more commonly used option for femoral shortening osteotomy is a subtrochanteric osteotomy. This is generally my preferred option. It allows for preservation of the metaphyseal region for implant fixation and eliminates the need for a greater trochanteric osteotomy. However, it is more technically challenging, and nonunion of the osteotomy site can still occur. It also requires more extensive soft-tissue dissection of the proximal femur in order to expose the subtrochanteric region, although as much as possible of the femoral soft-tissue attachments with their vascularity should be preserved to promote osteotomy healing. Several options are available for subtrochanteric osteotomies. Step-cut, oblique, or simple transverse osteotomies can be performed. I prefer transverse osteotomies because they are easier to perform, and they allow rotational abnormalities to

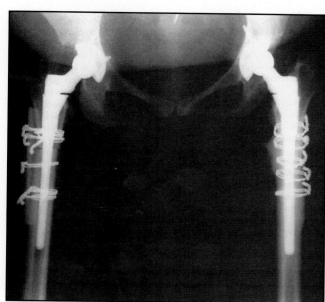

Figure 18-1. The x-ray demonstrates bilateral total hip replacements with subtrochanteric osteotomies fixed with wires and supplemental cortical grafts. There has been incorporation of the graft on the left side. (Reproduced with permission from Rorabeck CH, Burnett RSJ. Total hip arthroplasty: high hip dislocation. In: Lieberman JR, Berry DJ, eds. *Advanced Reconstruction Hip.* Rosemont, IL: American Academy of Orthopaedic Surgeons; 2005:121-129.)

be corrected more readily. It is advisable to initially resect a little less bone than is planned from preoperative templating because additional bone can be resected if necessary.

Firm osteotomy fixation is necessary for healing and for rotational control of the femoral implant. Fixation of the osteotomy site is achieved with tight diaphyseal fixation of the stem in the distal fragment, often combined with a cortical graft. I prefer to augment with a graft to ensure adequate fixation when possible (Figure 18-1). The potential for some restoration of bone stock makes allograft preferable to supplemental plate fixation. Cortical allograft or autograft, which can sometimes be fashioned from the patient's resected bone, should be secured to the femur using 2 to 4 cerclage wires or cables. I prefer wires due to decreased fretting compared with cables. Several commercially available wire passers with thick gauge wires can be used. Alternatively, thinner wires can be doubled over, passed around the femur, and tightened with heavy pliers or more conventional wire-tightening devices. If this technique is used, the wires should be passed twice around the femur and then tightened, rather than simply folded over and passed a single time before tightening, because the frictional forces will be much higher allowing for greater compression of the graft to the osteotomy site and more rigid fixation (Figure 18-2). It is advisable to ensure the soft tissue envelope of the femur will close over the construct before final tightening, especially in smaller patients.

In addition to the normal postoperative management of a total hip replacement patient, these patients should be carefully assessed for sciatic nerve function and the need for a shoe lift. The reconstruction should be protected from full weightbearing for at least 3 months to monitor union of the osteotomy site.

Figure 18-2. Wire A was passed, as described in the text, by passing it around the femur twice and then tightened. Wire B was simply folded in half and passed a single time. The techniques used for Wire A will provide greater fixation due to the increase in frictional forces.

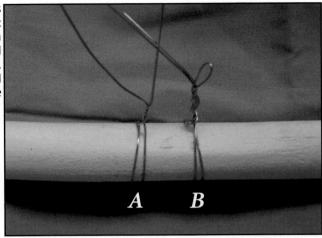

A   B

References

1. Crowe JF, Mani VJ, Ranawat CS. Total hip replacement in congenital dislocation and dysplasia of the hip. *J Bone Joint Surg Am.* 1979;61(1):15–23.
2. Sanchez-Sotelo J, Trousdale RT, Berry DJ, Cabanela ME. Surgical treatment of developmental dysplasia of the hip in adults: I. Nonarthroplasty options. *J Am Acad Orthop Surg.* 2002;10(5):321–333.
3. Lewallen DG. Neurovascular injury associated with hip arthroplasty. *Instr Course Lect.* 1998;47:275–283.

I Have a Patient With Start-Up Thigh Pain 5 Years After Surgery, and I Think the Femoral Component Is Loose. How Can I Tell for Sure?

Calin S. Moucha, MD

Thigh pain 5 years after a total hip replacement can be caused by a variety of conditions. Although aseptic loosening is always a possibility, extrinsic and other intrinsic causes of pain must always be ruled out.

I first like to rule out the extrinsic causes of pain. Thigh pain with tenderness over the greater trochanter may be caused by trochanteric bursitis. Local anesthetic injection into the trochanteric bursa administered with a form of steroid is both diagnostic and therapeutic. Spine disease, such as thoracolumbar discogenic pain, L3-4 posterior-lateral disc herniations or L4-5 foraminal disc herniations, may also cause groin and thigh pain, with or without associated low back pain. As such, I like to do a thorough back examination to rule out such conditions.

A loose femoral component often causes "start-up" pain: anterior thigh pain or knee pain that worsens with ambulation. Perhaps due to the component obtaining a stable position within the femoral canal, this pain often subsides with prolonged ambulation. On occasion, patients may present with an external rotation contracture due to the loose femoral component rotating into retroversion. Subjective feelings of the hip "giving out" may also be associated with a loose femoral component. This is most likely related to shortening of the limb and associated decrease in soft-tissue tension at the level of the hip joint.

During the physical exam of a patient with a loose femoral component, I commonly observe an antalgic gait caused by motion of the stem within the femoral canal. With significant stem subsidence, I often see an abductor lurch: as the abductors shorten they are at a biomechanical disadvantage. I have on occasion measured limb-length discrepancies,

Figure 19-1. Preoperative roentgenogram of a symptomatic patient 3 years after total hip replacement. Note endosteal scalloping, generalized osteolysis, and cortical hypertrophy. Intraoperative cultures confirmed prosthetic joint infection.

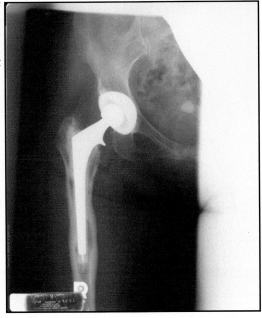

with the affected side being shorter. I find my patients rarely complain of this shortening, as it most likely occurred over a long period of time and they have gotten used to it. Many patients who have loose femoral components experience thigh pain when asked to perform an active straight leg raise in the supine position. Passive internal and external rotation of the hip joint occasionally causes thigh pain, but not always. Vastus lateralis muscle herniation through a defect in the fascia lata is an unusual cause of thigh pain that has been described. This can be palpated as a mass when the muscle is tensed.

Infection as the cause of pain after total hip replacement must always be ruled out. Pain while at rest, night pain, fevers, chills, recent dental procedures, other hip procedures prior to the hip replacement, or prolonged wound drainage after the index procedure all raise my suspicion for infection. These patients often have radiographs that show endosteal scalloping, generalized osteolysis, and periosteal new bone formation (Figure 19-1). I like to check a complete blood count with differential (CBC), erythrocyte sedimentation rate (ESR), and a C-reactive protein (CRP). If any of these values are elevated and the patient does not have other sources of infection, I will aspirate the hip under fluoroscopic guidance.

To make the diagnosis of a loose femoral component, I rely predominantly on plain radiographs. I routinely obtain a standard anterior posterior (AP) pelvic radiograph and AP, frog lateral, and cross-table lateral of the affected hip. Digital radiographs allow quality optimization so that the interface between the bone and prosthesis, cement and prosthesis, or cement and bone can be visualized. Standard radiographs that patients bring in themselves must be less than a week old and be of sufficient quality to be used for evaluation. As radiographic signs are often subtle and progress slowly, comparison of serial radiographs is critical in the evaluation of a prosthetic joint replacement. My staff spends a great deal of energy assisting patients in the process of obtaining these films.

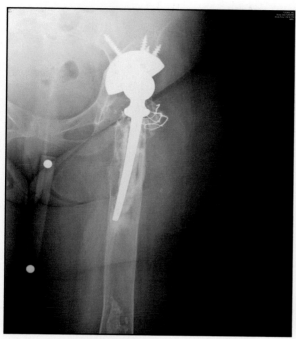

Figure 19-2. Preoperative roentgenogram of a symptomatic patient 15 years after total hip replacement and 3 years after revision of the acetabular component. Note circumferential radiolucencies, cortical discontinuity, and cement fracture. Gross loosening was confirmed intraoperatively.

I assess the stability of cemented and cementless implants using different criteria. For cemented femoral implants, especially those designed to bond to the cement mantle, I look for radiolucent lines at the prosthesis-cement interface suggestive of debonding. I then evaluate the bone-cement interface. One of the following findings indicates to me "definite" component loosening: migration of the component, fracture of the stem, or cement fracture. A continuous radiolucent line at the bone-cement interface (Figure 19-2) that is greater than 2 mm in width tells me that the component is "probably loose." When that line is present between 50% and 100% of the total bone-cement interface, the stem is "possibly loose." When old radiographs are available for review, the "probably loose" and the "possibly loose" implants become "definitely loose" if these lines are progressive. If the radiolucencies just described were present on radiographs taken soon after the surgery, or if these early radiographs are not available for evaluation, I order a technetium 99 methylene diphosphonate scan. If the scan reveals normal findings, I continue my search for extrinsic causes of hip pain. If the scan is positive and it has been more than 2 years since the surgery was done, I discuss revision surgery with the patient.

In patients who have had their hip replacement done many years prior to their evaluation, I interpret radiolucent lines at the femoral bone-cement interface with more caution than in those who have had their surgery done more recently. In these generally older patients, radiolucent lines may indicate internal bone remodeling rather than loosening at the bone-cement interface.

I assess cementless femoral components using different criteria (Figures 19-3 and 19-4). Regardless of fixation zone (proximal or distal), the presence of progressive implant migration on serial radiographs is highly suggestive of implant loosening. On the other hand, absence of reactive lines or presence of "endosteal" spot welds around the porous-coated part of the prosthesis are highly consistent with a well-fixed implant.

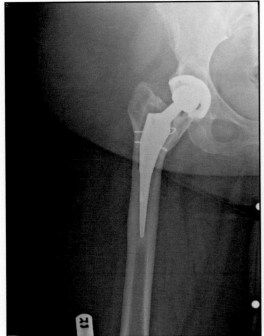

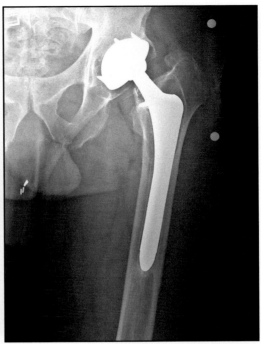

Figure 19-3. Preoperative roentgenogram 6 years after placement of a cementless proximally fixed tapered stem. Note subsidence, radiolucent lines, and formation of a pedestal. Gross loosening was confirmed intraoperatively.

Figure 19-4. Preoperative roentgenogram 7 years after placement of a fully coated cementless stem. Note subsidence, bead shedding, radiolucent lines, lack of spot welds, and early pedestal formation.

Visualizing spot welds on proximally porous-coated implants or on extensively coated implants that are canal filling is often difficult. As such, I also look for other "minor" signs of osseointegration. These include calcar atrophy, the absence of bead shedding, and the absence of a pedestal. Pedestals without associated radiolucent stems, however, must be interpreted with caution—they are not always indicative of loosening. Cortical hypertrophy proximally in a collared implant may indicate loosening, whereas cortical hypertrophy distally in a fully coated implant is suggestive of osseointegration. As with cemented implants, it is rare that I use nuclear imaging to evaluate a patient's femoral component. On the rare occasion that I obtain these tests, however, I interpret them with caution, especially when the results are abnormal.

Diagnosing a loose femoral component is not always easy. Although other techniques such as fluoroscopy, arthrography, and dynamic computerized tomography have been evaluated in the scientific literature, I rarely find these tests necessary. Currently, I find comparison of serial radiographs to be the most useful method for making the appropriate diagnosis. When loosening, infection, and extrinsic causes of hip pain have been ruled out, other causes of thigh pain must be worked up. These include mismatch in the modulus of elasticity between an implant and host bone, stress fractures, and oncological processes.

Bibliography

Engh CA, Massin P, Suthers KE. Roentgenographic assessment of the biologic fixation of porous-surfaced femoral components. *Clin Orthop Relat Res.* 1990;257;107-128.

Higgs JE, Chong A, Haertsch P, Sekel R, Leicester A. An unusual cause of thigh pain after total hip arthroplasty. *J Arthroplasty.* 1995;10(2):203-204.

O'Neill DA, Harris WH. Failed total hip replacement: assessment by plain radiographs, arthrograms, and aspiration of the hip joint. *J Bone Joint Surg Am.* 1984;66(4):540-546.

Tehranzadeh J, Schneider R, Freiberger RH. Radiological evaluation of painful total hip replacement. *Radiology.* 1981;141(2):355-362.

I HAVE A PATIENT WITH A LARGE AMOUNT OF FEMORAL OFFSET. HOW DO I ADDRESS THIS INTRAOPERATIVELY?

Matthew Beal, MD
Kirstina Olson, MD
David Manning, MD

Femoral offset is defined as the perpendicular distance from the anatomic axis of the femur to the hip joint center of rotation. Large femoral offset is commonly encountered in male patients, large patients, patients with coxa vara, and in those patients with previous slipped capital femoral epiphysis. Failure to maintain native femoral offset in such patients undergoing total hip arthroplasty (THA) has several deleterious effects, including loss of abductor power, decreased bearing performance, and instability.

A loss of femoral offset after THA decreases abductor power by diminishing the abductor moment arm. In some cases, the loss of abductor power may result in prolonged limp after THA. In addition, decreased abductor moment arm results in an increased joint reaction force, which has a negative impact on bearing stress and bearing wear performance. Sakalkale et al have shown in a group of patients with bilateral hip replacements that the linear wear rate in hips with standard-offset femoral components was 0.21 mm/yr as compared with an average of 0.01 mm/yr for hips with high-offset components at 5 years. Other clinical investigations have shown that when femoral offset is maintained after a THA, there are beneficial effects on gait, including optimized abductor function, decreased incidence of Trendelenburg gait, and decreased dependence on walking aids. What is most apparent intraoperatively during THA is that failure to restore femoral offset commonly results in instability from femoral-pelvic impingement in positions of combined hyperextension-external rotation, as well as combined flexion-adduction-internal rotation.

A patient's natural offset and neck-shaft angle can be evaluated using standard anterior posterior (AP) pelvis and AP hip radiographs. Templating these radiographs allows us to detect high offset situations preoperatively and plan accordingly. There are several ways to introduce femoral offset intraoperatively when performing a THA. Increasing the neck length will increase offset along with the potentially deleterious effect of increasing leg length. Most THA systems address offset in an isolated fashion by providing a femoral component option with increased offset. Systems achieve increased offset through the femoral component by either offering a lateralized neck option or a decreased neck-shaft angle option. The components are normalized to leg length so that intraoperative trialing of these options does not have an effect on leg length. A high-offset femoral component is always our first option when addressing the high-offset hip. If further offset is required, extended offset polyethylene liner and head options are available. The offset liner achieves increased offset via augmented material thickness at the pole of the articulation. Lateralizing the hip center through the use of an offset liner is our second preference when addressing the high-offset hip due to the detrimental effects of increased body moment arm, joint reaction force, bearing stress, and wear. The offset femoral head option involves an eccentric morse taper location on the femoral ball, allowing it to be placed eccentrically on the neck. We prefer not to use this option, as it results in increased torsional forces on the head-neck junction, potentially increasing fretting.

When preoperative templating predicts that high-offset femoral components in combination with offset liner options will fail to restore preoperative offset, as a last option, we choose to position the acetabular component slightly lateral to the medial wall of the pelvis. In these types of cases, instead of using my initial reamer to identify the medial wall, we establish my new hip center within the medial wall osteophyte. This is demonstrated in the case example seen in Figures 20-1 and 20-2. A small drill and depth gauge can be used to measure the lateral distance from the medial wall to match any need identified during preoperative templating. We use this technique as a last resort, and would, as a rule, recommend always medializing the acetabular component to the teardrop to maximize prosthetic surface area contact with host bone and minimize joint reactive force.

Our greatest tool in managing the high-offset hip is preoperative templating and planning. When preoperative templating is not routinely performed, and the high-offset scenario is not predicted, the first indication may be intraoperative instability. If instability is encountered, and the acetabular and femoral components are confirmed to be in appropriate position, this is an offset problem. The greater trochanter may act as a fulcrum and lever the femoral bearing from the acetabulum by impinging on the anterior pelvis in the position of flexion, adduction, and internal rotation or alternatively by impinging on the posterior pelvis in the position of hyperextension and external rotation. The unprepared surgeon is frequently relegated to managing the situation by simply increasing femoral neck length. The result is an unacceptable limb length inequality, postoperative limp, and an unsatisfied patient. In this scenario, the only option to preserve limb length equality may be to perform a trochanteric advancement.

At the beginning of each case, we perform an initial comparison of the relative leg lengths and compare it to our preoperative templated measurement of limb length. Both heels and knees should be aligned and palpable under the drapes, so a direct comparison can be made once the trial components are in place and again once the final components are implanted. Many techniques have been described to assess limb length intraoperatively and we recommend using several in each case, as no one method is completely accurate. We prefer to test stability in various positions including the position of sleep

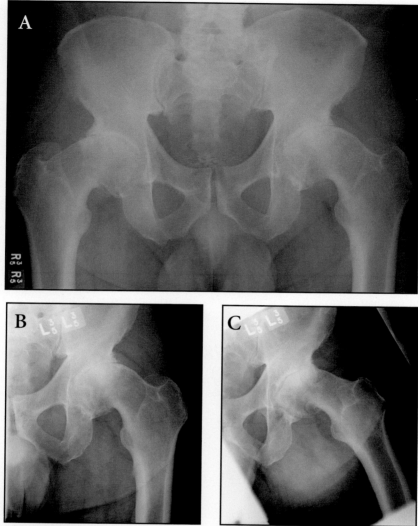

Figure 20-1. Anterior-posterior (AP) pelvic radiograph, AP hip radiograph, and lateral hip radiograph depicting bilateral osteoarthritis with evidence of old slipped capital femoral epiphysis. This is a high-offset situation with shortened, varus femoral necks. The patient is at increased risk for femoral–pelvic impingement, dislocation, and limb length inequality after THA.

(hip adducted 30 degrees, hip and knee flexed 30 degrees); 20 degrees hyperextension with maximal external rotation; full flexion; and flexion to 45 degrees and 90 degrees with measured internal rotation. When performing THA through a posterior lateral approach, my minimal acceptable stability in 45 degrees and 90 degrees of hip flexion is 70 degrees and 45 degrees internal rotation, respectively. Excellent stability, equal limb lengths, and optimal biomechanics are achievable in the high-offset hip when preoperative templating is coupled with the strategies outlined in this question.

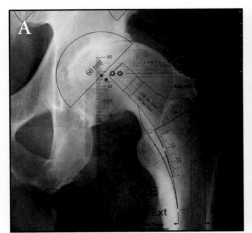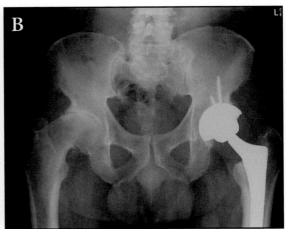

Figure 20-2. (A) Preoperative template of left hip reconstruction. Image depicts high-offset scenario in which templated reconstruction does not adequately restore preoperative offset despite 5-mm extended offset liner option, large extended offset stem, and short femoral neck cut. (B) Reconstruction with slightly lateralized acetabular component, 3.5-mm lateralized liner, large extended offset stem, and 0-mm head-neck combination. Result is equal limb lengths and 34.6 mm of reconstruction offset compared with 34.2 mm of native offset.

Bibliography

Sakalkale DP, Sharkey PF, Eng K, Hozack WJ, Rothman RH. Effect of femoral component offset on polyethylene wear in total hip arthroplasty. *Clin Orthop Relat Res.* 2001;(388):125-134.

I HAVE A PATIENT WITH AN INFECTED WELL-FIXED FEMORAL COMPONENT. HOW DO I REMOVE THIS WITHOUT DESTROYING THE FEMORAL BONE?

Brett Levine, MD, MS

Extraction of well-fixed femoral components in the setting of prosthetic hip infection requires significant preoperative planning, meticulous surgical technique, and appropriate postoperative care. The following question will discuss the approach I use in removing a well-fixed femoral implant after confirmation of prosthetic hip infection.

Preoperative Planning

Preoperative planning is a crucial aspect in safely removing a well-fixed femoral component. When possible, previous operative reports are obtained and components identified. A thorough history and physical is performed to evaluate for clinical evidence of component loosening, prior surgical incisions, and hip and knee contractures.

Appropriate preoperative radiographs are evaluated to identify the type of femoral component and determine where and how fixation to the femur is achieved. Further considerations include evidence of component loosening, grade of cement mantle, and surrounding bone quality (Paprosky classification).[1-3]

Preoperative indications for an extended trochanteric osteotomy (ETO) include well-fixed fully coated stems, cemented stems with a long distal mantle, femoral varus remodeling, and precoated cemented stems. Planning includes templating an optimal length for the osteotomy so that component/cement removal is facilitated, while leaving sufficient (greater than 4 cm) distal femur for reimplantation.[4]

Figure 21-1. (A) Elevation of the vastus lateralis from the lateral intermuscular septum. (B) The osteotomy length is then measured from the tip of the greater trochanter distally to a preoperatively templated level.

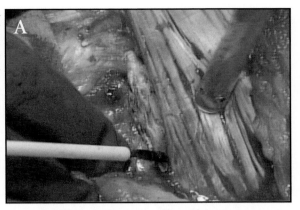

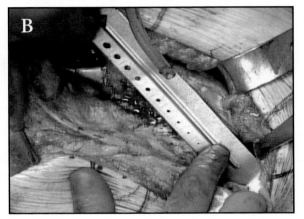

Surgical Technique

I use a standard posterior approach to the hip for revision surgery. After collection of intraoperative infection parameters is complete, gross stability of the component is assessed. Initial attempts are made to remove the femoral component in an atraumatic manner. For proximally coated cementless implants I use flexible osteotomes, pencil tip burrs, and/or a cementless ultrasound device to disrupt the implant-bone interface. When successful, standard extraction devices can be used to remove the implant. For cemented components with poor/short cement mantles and non-precoated stems, extraction of the component from above is straightforward after the visible cement is cleared proximally. I then remove the remaining cement mantle using a series of cement osteotomes, drills, and/or an ultrasound device.

In cases where an ETO is required, further exposure of the proximal femur is necessary. The vastus lateralis is elevated from the intramuscular septum along a preoperatively determined length (Figure 21-1). For proximally coated stems with distal bone ongrowth, an ETO must extend to the end of the porous coating. In cases where there is varus remodeling or an extensively coated implant has been used, the ETO is planned to afford a minimum of 4 cm of isthmic bone distally. With cemented implants, the osteotomy is planned to either the tip of the stem or cement plug.

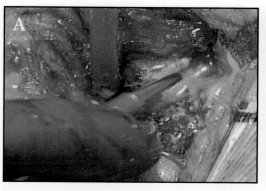 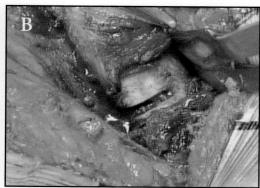

Figure 21-2. (A) The lateral femoral cortex is then marked with a burr distally and (B) the edges rounded to connect the anterior and posterior limbs of the osteotomy.

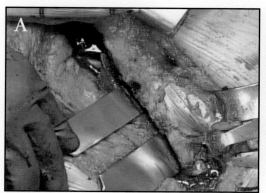 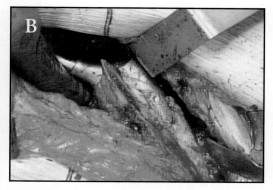

Figure 21-3. (A) Large straight osteotomes are used sequentially to elevate the osteotomy and create a controlled fracture along the anterior femoral cortex. (B) The osteotomy fragment is retracted anteriorly to give exposure to the femoral stem.

Care is taken during dissection to avoid inadvertent sectioning of the femoral perforators as adequate exposure is achieved. I then score the femur posteriorly using a pencil tip burr and mark the distal extent of the osteotomy laterally. The osteotomy edges are rounded and using the burr I extend proximally along the anterior cortex for the distance that is visible (Figure 21-2). I plan for removal of approximately one-third to one-half of the lateral aspect of the femur. An oscillating saw is utilized to complete the osteotomy posteriorly. When possible, cemented stems are removed prior to the osteotomy and the femur may be sectioned across to the anterior cortex. A series of wide straight osteotomes are then used to elevate the osteotomy fragment (Figure 21-3). This affords a controlled fracture of the anterior cortex and maintains a well-vascularized osteotomy fragment.[5,6]

The osteotomy fragment is retracted anteriorly and a Gigli's saw (have several of these available) or burr is used to disrupt the bone/cement-implant bond. Typically, the stem is easily extracted at this time. However, if an extensively coated stem is in place, it may be necessary to section the stem with a metal-cutting burr. Trephines are then used to ream over the distal stem and allow extraction of the remaining implant.

Once the component is safely extracted, a cerclage wire is placed distal to the osteotomy site and the femur is débrided with flexible reamers and curettes. My preference is to use

Figure 21-4. (A) Preoperative AP hip radiograph of an infected THA.

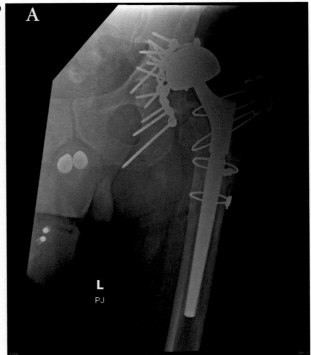

Luque wires or nonbraided cables to secure the osteotomy after a nonarticulating cement spacer is fashioned (Figure 21-4). Typically, 2 to 3 cables/wires are used to securely fix the osteotomy site. Care is taken to reapproximate the osteotomy edges without excessive tension. A gap at the distal extent of the osteotomy of up to 1 cm is acceptable.

Postoperative Care

Organism-specific antibiotics are used to treat the infection for a minimum of 6 weeks. Patients are allowed foot-flat weightbearing and are instructed to avoid active abduction if an ETO was required. Patients are assessed clinically at 2 and 6 weeks postoperatively for evidence of infection eradication.

Utilizing this method, I have been able to safely eradicate infection in the majority of my patients. A recently published report has shown an 87% rate of infection eradication in cases where an ETO was necessary for safe extraction of a well-fixed femoral component.[7] Reported osteotomy healing rates range between 96% to 100%, even in the face of infection.[8] Immediate fixation of the osteotomy at the first stage is not detrimental or associated with higher reinfection rates. It can however, afford an intact proximal femur, allowing insertion of smaller revision and primary components at the time reimplantation.

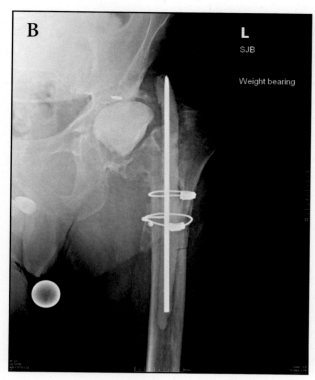

Figure 21-4. (B) AP hip radiograph after ETO, removal of the prosthesis, and placement of a cement spacer. (C) Postoperative radiograph after infection eradication and reimplantation.

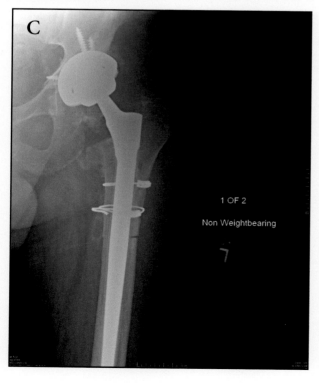

Conclusion

* Obtain prior operative reports.
* Preoperative plan (identify components, ETO, operating room equipment).
* Attempt atraumatic implant extraction.
* Indications for ETO:
  * Well-fixed extensively coated implant
  * Long distal cement mantle
  * Varus remodeling of femur
  * Precoated cemented stems
* Secure fixation of ETO at time of spacer placement.

References

1. Valle CJ, Paprosky WG. Classification and an algorithmic approach to the reconstruction of femoral deficiency in revision total hip arthroplasty. *J Bone Joint Surg Am.* 2003;85-A(Suppl 4):1-6.
2. Engh CA, Massin P, Suthers KE. Roentgenographic assessment of the biologic fixation of porous-surfaced femoral components. *Clin Orthop Relat Res.* 1990;257:107-128.
3. Harris WH, McGann WA. Loosening of the femoral component after use of the medullary-plug cementing technique: follow-up note with a minimum five-year follow-up. *J Bone Joint Surg Am.* 1986;68(7):1064-1066.
4. Paprosky WG, Aribindi R. Hip replacement: treatment of femoral bone loss using distal bypass fixation. *Instr Course Lect.* 2000;49:119-130.
5. Paprosky WG, Sporer SM. Controlled femoral fracture: easy in. *J Arthroplasty.* 2003;18(3 Suppl 1):91-93.
6. Younger TI, Bradford MS, Magnus RE, Paprosky WG. Extended proximal femoral osteotomy: a new technique for femoral revision arthroplasty. *J Arthroplasty.* 1995;10(3):329-338.
7. Levine B, Della Valle CJ, Hamming M, Sporer S, Berger RA, Paprosky W. Use of extended trochanteric osteotomy in treating prosthetic hip infection. *J Arthroplasty.* 2008; April 8 [epub ahead of print].
8. Morshed S, Huffman GR, Ries MD. Extended trochanteric osteotomy for 2-stage revision of infected total hip arthroplasty. *J Arthroplasty.* 2005;20(3):294-301.

I HAVE A PATIENT WITH A LOOSE FEMORAL COMPONENT AND VARUS REMODELING OF THE PROXIMAL FEMUR. WHAT SURGICAL APPROACH AND IMPLANT SHOULD I USE?

Stephen M. Walsh, MD, FRCSC

The overall approach to any hip revision requires careful and thoughtful preoperative planning. A detailed history and physical examination are mandatory. In addition, obtaining prior operative reports and implant records is invaluable. Anticipating pitfalls such as poor visualization, instability, and component integrity will greatly alleviate intraoperative stress when such situations arise. It is important to consider the cause of failure and to rule out infection through appropriate laboratory analysis and aspiration.

I employ a posterior approach when revising total hips. The posterior approach is extensible for both femoral and acetabular reconstruction. It is often necessary to re-create soft tissue planes, which can be facilitated by extending the incision beyond the original scar. I start by identifying the fascia lata and fascia of the gluteus maximus and raising full-thickness skin flaps. The fascial layer is divided inline with the incision and freed from the gluteus medius and vastus lateralis. The sciatic nerve is palpated and protected; however, it is rarely necessary to directly free the nerve. Identification of the posterior border of the medius can be difficult. The posterior border of the greater trochanter is an excellent landmark in this case. Extensive release of the pseudocapsule is paramount prior to attempting dislocation to decrease risk of fracture.

It is very tempting to immediately remove a loose stem after dislocation. To avoid fracture, first remove any soft tissue, overgrown bone, or cement covering the superolateral corner of the stem. In the presence of varus remodeling, it may not be possible to remove the stem without an osteotomy.

The extended trochanteric osteotomy greatly facilitates femoral revision under a variety of circumstances. These may include a well-fixed cemented or cementless stem, the

Figure 22-1. Anterior-posterior (AP) hip x-ray displaying a loose stem and varus remodeling. The overlying revision stem template highlights the utility of the extended trochanteric osteotomy in canal preparation and deformity correction.

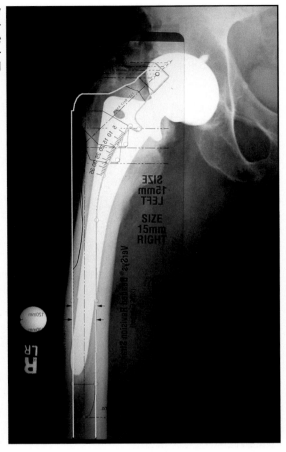

presence of distal cement, varus or torsional remodeling, difficult acetabular exposure, and extensive trochanteric lysis.[1,2] The presence of varus remodeling may inhibit stem removal and can make femoral canal preparation and reimplantation nearly impossible (Figure 22-1). Osteotomy will allow direct access to the distal canal and correction of deformity.

The basic steps of the extended trochanteric osteotomy are creation, elevation, and fixation (Figure 22-2). The osteotomy may be performed prior to dislocation, with the implant in place, or after implant removal (preferred). The osteotomized fragment includes the greater trochanter and the lateral one-third of the proximal femoral cortex. It is extended as needed to allow implant removal or deformity correction with a minimum distance from the greater trochanter of about 12 cm, or enough to allow fixation with 2 cables. In the presence of varus remodeling, proper preoperative templating will identify the point of maximal deformity and this typically dictates the distal extent of the osteotomy. Posteriorly, the osteotomy extends from the posterior greater trochanter along the linea aspera posterior to the vastus lateralis. The gluteus maximus tendon is released as needed for femoral mobilization. An oscillating saw or pencil tip burr is employed for the posterior cut. To avoid a stress riser, the pencil tip burr is utilized to round off the corners of the osteotomy. Ideally, prior implant removal allows a through and through cut with a

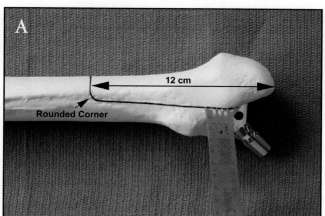

Figure 22-2. (A) Posterior osteotomy line displaying rounded distal corner and transverse component 12 cm from the tip of the greater trochanter. (B) Anterior osteotomy line proximal and distal to guide controlled fracture. (C) Elevation of osteotomized fragment with multiple broad osteotomes.

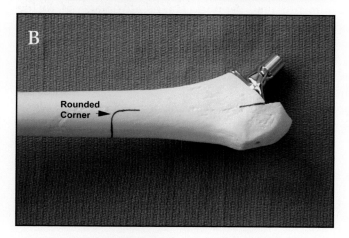

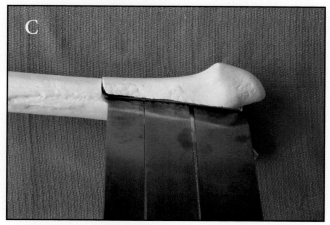

completely free fragment. When the implant remains, the vastus lateralis is mobilized to allow the anterior osteotomy line to extend from distal to proximal for 2 to 3 cm. Proximally, the anterior osteotomy is started at the anterior edge of the greater trochanter for 1 to 2 cm. This guides a controlled fracture as the fragment is carefully and slowly elevated with multiple broad osteotomes. The intact attachments of the gluteus medius and vastus lateralis maintain blood supply and soft tissue balance.

I place a cable just distal to the osteotomy to help avoid fracture propagation if a stress riser has been created. The canal side of the osteotomized fragment is machined with a high-speed barrel burr to accommodate the lateral geometry of the stem. When closing the osteotomy, I rotate the fragment posteriorly to tightly close any posterior gap. This allows adequate surface area for healing and helps to avoid anterior bony impingement of the greater trochanter. The tension of the gluteus medius may be increased by translating the greater trochanter distally. Fixation typically requires 2 or 3 cables.

Implant choice varies with defect and deformity. Varus remodeling addressed with an extended trochanteric osteotomy typically is treated with a distally fixed implant. Choices may include an extensively porous-coated cylindrical stem (either straight or curved) or a modular tapered revision stem. These stems obtain a tight scratch fit in the distal isthmus and do not require proximal support. This is advantageous in the presence of proximal bone loss or deformity. It is necessary to obtain a scratch fit over 4 to 6 cm when a cylindrical stem is employed. The stem itself must have adequate strength to endure cyclic loading as there is a risk of implant fracture in the absence of proximal bony support. Reported results for femoral revision with extensively coated stems reveal low rates of mechanical failure.[3,4]

Postoperatively, patients are kept partial weight bearing for 8 to 12 weeks to allow ample time for osteotomy healing and bony integration of the stem.

References

1. Younger TI, Bradford MS, Magnus RE, Paprosky WG. Extended proximal femoral osteotomy: a new technique for femoral revision arthroplasty. *J Arthroplasty*. 1995;10(3):329-338.
2. Meek RMD, Greidanus NV, Garbuz DS, Masri BA, Duncan CP. Extended trochanteric osteotomy: planning, surgical technique, and pitfalls. *Instr Course Lect*. 2004;53:119-130.
3. Krishnamurthy AB, MacDonald SJ, Paprosky WG. 5- to 13-year follow-up study on cementless components in revision surgery. *J Arthroplasty*. 1997;12(8):839-847.
4. Engh CA, Hopper RH, Engh CA. Distal ingrowth components. *Clin Orthop Relat Res*. 2004;420:135-141.

I Have a Patient With Distal Osteolysis and a Loose Stem. What Type of Implant Should I Use and What Bone Stock Can I Anticipate Finding at the Time of Surgery?

Mark F. Schinsky, MD

When preparing for a revision total hip arthroplasty, bony deficiencies must be accurately assessed and classified to ensure proper treatment choices. Several classification systems have been described for femoral defects, including the system developed by the American Academy of Orthopaedic Surgeons Committee on the Hip, the Endo-Klinik classification, the Mallory classification, the Saleh system, and the Paprosky femoral defect classification.

The Paprosky classification system provides an algorithmic approach to femoral assessment based on the location and extent of bone loss and helps guide the surgeon in selecting the appropriate method for reconstruction. The surgeon must use both the preoperative radiographs as well as the intraoperative findings to properly assess the femoral bone quality. Once the existing femoral component has been removed, a reverse hook curette can be used to sound the femoral canal, remove any existing pseudomembrane, and ensure previously used cement has been entirely removed. This intraoperative technique may reveal bone loss or defects in the patient's host bone that was unsuspected on preoperative radiographs alone. The Paprosky femoral defect classification system can then be applied to these assessments, arranging the deficiencies into 5 basic types as follows[1,2]:

1. Type I: In Type I defects, bone loss is minimal and primarily of the cancellous metaphyseal bone with only partial loss of the calcar and anterior posterior (AP) bone. The diaphysis remains intact. This type of bone loss can be seen in

resurfacings or after removal of a cementless femoral component without a biologic ingrowth surface. Femora with these defects are not significantly different
from those seen during primary total hip arthroplasty.

2. Type II: In Type II defects, the diaphysis remains intact; however, the calcar is
   deficient with extensive metaphyseal cancellous bone loss. These defects are
   often seen after severe femoral component subsidence, metaphyseal osteolysis, or
   removal of a cemented component.

3. Type IIIA: In Type IIIA defects, the metaphysis is severely damaged and the defect
   involves the junction with the diaphysis. In this defect type, a minimum of 4 cm of
   scratch-fit can be obtained near the isthmus. This defect type can be encountered
   after removal of a grossly loose cemented femoral component that was put in with
   first-generation cement techniques.

4. Type IIIB: In Type IIIB defects, the metaphysis is severely damaged and the defect
   extends further into the diaphysis with less than 4 cm of diaphyseal bone available for distal fixation. Distal osteolysis seen with cementless femoral prostheses
   or failed cemented components inserted using cement restrictors can lead to this
   type of defect.

5. Type IV: In Type IV defects, both the metaphysis and the diaphysis are extensively
   damaged, the cortices are thinned with a widened femoral canal, and the isthmus
   is nonsupportive. These defects are rare but represent a significant challenge to
   reconstruct.

After the femoral bone loss is thoroughly assessed and the appropriate Paprosky femoral defect type determined, reconstruction can proceed. Reconstruction of a Type I defect
can proceed similar to a primary total hip arthroplasty (THA). Implant choices include
proximally porous-coated stems, 6-inch extensively coated stems, and cemented stems.
Intraoperative axial and rotational stability must be achieved.

As Type II defects lack supportive proximal bone and often have minimal remaining
cancellous bone, proximally porous-coated and cemented stems are generally not appropriate for reconstructing these femurs. Fully porous-coated stems that achieve distal fixation and bypass the proximal defect are preferred. A standard 6-inch stem can be used in
most patients, though a calcar replacement may be required.

Since Type IIIA defects retain at least 4 cm of diaphysis near the isthmus available for
a scratch-fit, an extensively porous-coated stem is an appropriate choice for reconstruction. These femora generally require the stem to be 8 or 10 inches in length to achieve
fixation. The anterior bow of the femur must be taken into consideration during reaming
and implant positioning. A bowed stem may be necessary to avoid perforation. Other
choices for reconstruction include impaction grafting or modular, cementless, distally
tapered stems.

Type IIIB defects often lack the diaphyseal bone necessary for successful placement of
cylindrical, extensively porous-coated implants. This implant design had a 50% failure
rate in one series when used for Type IIIB defects.[2] Even with a short isthmus, modular, cementless, distally tapered stems with flutes can achieve excellent initial axial and
rotational stability and are the implant of choice for these defects. The proximal modularity allows for alterations in limb length, offset, and femoral anteversion. Should the
cortical tube remain intact and the canal width exceed 18 mm, impaction grafting can

be undertaken. Impaction grafting involves cementing in a polished, tapered stem into a bed of firmly packed allograft. Potential advantages include improving the cancellous bed to accept cement in order to create a mechanically stable construct and restoring bone stock.

Options for reconstructing Type IV defects include impaction grafting, allograft prosthetic composites (APCs), and proximal femoral-replacing endoprostheses. The patient's age, activity level, and comorbidities help the surgeon choose the appropriate reconstruction. APCs can potentially restore bone stock, provide proximal support for the prosthesis, and allow for soft tissue and greater trochanter reattachment. APCs are generally reserved for younger patients. In elderly patients with lower activity levels or those patients who can not tolerate a more extensive procedure and have a nonreconstructable proximal femur, a femoral replacing endoprosthesis is an acceptable alternative.

Not every case can be precisely classified by any system, and multiple reconstruction options exist. However, the Paprosky femoral defect classification allows for an algorithmic, step-wise approach to the assessment of bony deficiencies and their ultimate reconstruction.

References

1. Paprosky WG, Burnett RS. Assessment and classification of bone stock deficiency in revision total hip arthroplasty. *Am J Orthop.* 2002;31(8):459.
2. Della Valle CJ, Paprosky WG. Classification and an algorithmic approach to the reconstruction of femoral deficiency in revision total hip arthroplasty. *J Bone Joint Surg Am.* 2003;85-A(Supp 4):1.

AN 84-YEAR-OLD MALE WHO HAD A PREVIOUS CEMENTED TOTAL HIP REPLACEMENT WITH SEVERE PROXIMAL OSTEOLYSIS FELL AND HAS A PERIPROSTHETIC FEMUR FRACTURE. HE HAS VERY LITTLE PROXIMAL BONE. SHOULD I RECONSTRUCT THIS WITH ALLOGRAFT BONE OR USE A TUMOR PROSTHESIS?

John L. Masonis, MD
Thomas K. Fehring, MD

This case includes multiple challenges: cement removal, fracture fixation, revision implant fixation, bone loss surrounding the greater trochanter, and postoperative stability.

The Vancouver classification system for periprosthetic femur fractures describes the location of the fracture, stability of the femoral component, and the bone quality.[1] This case represents a Vancouver B3 fracture. The fracture is at the level of the stem, the stem is loose, and the proximal bone is deficient (Figure 24-1).

It is important to have full length anterior-posterior (AP) and lateral femur films when reviewing the preoperative radiographs to evaluate the extent of the fracture and distal fixation options (Figure 24-2). It is also important to evaluate the acetabular component for loosening, wear, and modularity. If the cup is well fixed, well positioned, and modular, it is important to know what liner options are available at the time of revision.

Figure 24-1. Vancouver B3 fracture.

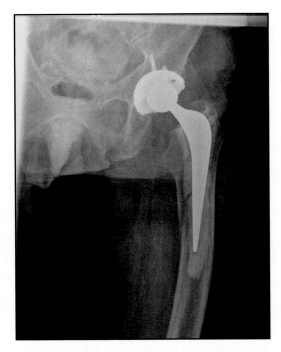

Figure 24-2. Distal femoral radiograph.

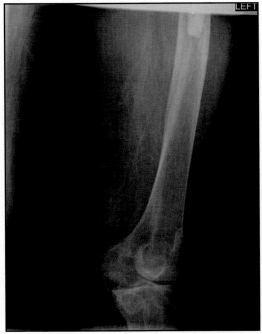

Specifically, you need to know if a larger diameter liner is available and if a constrained liner option is available. We try to use the biggest head available for revisions in this elderly age group. This is important because of the high rates of dislocation following revision total hip arthroplasty (THA).[2] If the acetabular component is well positioned and stable but does not have a "modern" modular polyethylene option, the inner diameter of the cup is evaluated for potential cementation of a new liner. This requires knowledge of the polyethylene outer diameter to ensure a minimum 2-mm cement mantle.

We prefer to utilize an extensile posterolateral approach for exposure that allows access for acetabular revision, preservation of the abductors, and unlimited distal femoral exposure with preservation of the vastus innervation. We treat the proximal fragment as you would a trochanteric slide osteotomy to aid in exposure and preserve the abductor insertion. It is important to expose and work through the fracture site for cement removal.

Cement removal can be performed using hand instruments or a high-speed burr by working through the fracture site and trochanteric slide. If remaining distal cement is well fixed, an ultrasonic device is used for cement removal.

The key consideration in decision making is the quality of proximal bone stock and the presence or absence of a functioning diaphysis for fixation. In this particular case, the proximal bone stock is very deficient and the fracture extends into the diaphysis. The remaining intact diaphysis is <3 cm long before it begins to flare into metaphyseal bone. This case is similar to any Type IV femoral defect where the proximal bone is deficient and there is not enough diaphysis available for press-fit fixation.

At our center we try to maintain the proximal cortical bone and trochanter at all costs to help preserve stability postoperatively. We have found that the use of a proximal femoral implant or an allograft prosthetic composite mandates the use of a constrained implant in this age group. If the existing cup incorporates this design, it is used; if not, a constrained device is cemented into place. The caveat here is that the inner diameter must be large enough to accommodate an adequate cement mantle.

Since we try to avoid tumor prostheses and allograft prosthetic composites, the remaining options include a cemented long stem, impaction grafting, or a tapered splined distally fixed implant. We have reported excellent results with press-fit fully porous-coated implants "potted" into diaphysis when proximal bone is extremely deficient.[3] However, this technique requires an adequate amount of intact femoral diaphysis. Since the fracture in this case extended into the diaphysis and the remaining intact diaphysis was <3 cm, this was not an option.

In this age group a cemented long stem is a reasonable option. However, pressurization is difficult in long stems especially with coexisting fractures. Therefore, we treated this case as we do most femoral reconstructions with Type IV femoral defects (ie, with a tapered modular implant).

Following cement removal, we prefer to reduce the fracture and use cables for fixation. Placing a slightly undersized femoral trial stem in the canal after cement removal and passage of cables can aid in diaphyseal reduction. We prefer to leave the trochanteric fragment mobile during femoral preparation. In addition, one cable should be placed 2 cm distal to the site of tapered fixation to prevent iatrogenic extension of the fracture when reaming or impacting the stem. Conical reaming of the diaphyseal bone is completed until cortical contact is solid. Proximal modular body reconstruction is then performed to restore femoral length.

Trial reductions are performed to evaluate hip stability and leg length. Head diameter should be maximized to reduce postoperative instability. Offset options are used to restore proximal femoral mechanics and reduce instability.

Fixation of the greater trochanteric fragment is difficult due to the proximal bone deficiency. We prefer to preserve the gluteus medius-vastus soft tissue sleeve and utilize

Figure 24-3. Tapered diaphyseal fixation stem and trochanteric cable plate.

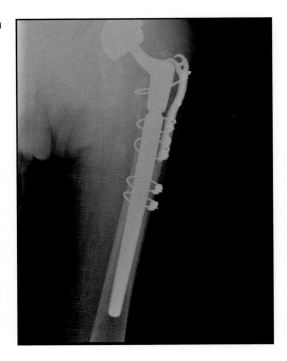

trochanteric cable plate fixation when proximal ingrowth is not expected because the plate requires fairly extensive stripping. Trochanteric wires can also be used when an extended trochanteric osteotomy has been used. With either technique, it is important to obtain transverse fixation through the plate below the lesser trochanter to prevent proximal migration of the plate as well as a wire running from just below the lesser trochanter obliquely in a cephalad direction around the body of the greater trochanter (Figure 24-3). Severe cortical bone loss of the proximal femur can be augmented with cortical strut allograft to prevent cable wire penetration of the weak proximal bone.

If the abductor deficiency is severe and the hip remains unstable despite maximizing the head diameter and liner options, then a constrained liner should be selected (Figure 24-4). It is important to recognize that constrained liner designs limit hip range of motion and transfer stress to the acetabular component-bone interface. Therefore, they should not be used indiscriminately.

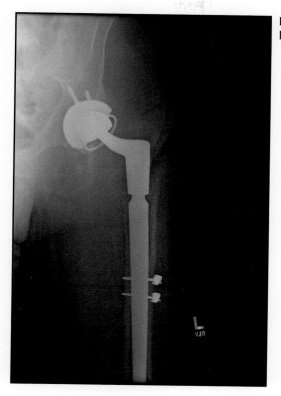

Figure 24-4. Revision stem with constrained liner and absent trochanter.

References

1. Brady OH, Garbuz DS, Masri BA, Duncan CP. Classification of the hip. *Orthop Clin North Am.* 1999;30(2):215-220.
2. Mulay S, Hassan T, Birtwistle S, Power R. Management of types B2 and B3 femoral periprosthetic fractures by a tapered, fluted, and distally fixed stem. *J Arthroplasty.* 2005;20(6):751-756.
3. Nadaud MC, Griffin WL, Fehring TK, et al. Cementless revision total hip arthroplasty without allograft in severe proximal femoral defects. *J Arthroplasty.* 2005;20(6):738-744.

SECTION IV

INTRAOPERATIVE GENERAL QUESTIONS

I WAS PLACING SCREWS IN THE ACETABULAR COMPONENT WHEN I BEGAN TO EXPERIENCE PROFUSE BLEEDING. WHAT SHOULD I DO?

Scott M. Sporer, MD

Vascular injuries following revision acetabular surgery are relatively rare, yet the potential consequence of major hemorrhage and subsequent death remain catastrophic. Vascular injuries observed during the surgical procedure occur most frequently while placing screws in the acetabular component or during the removal of an acetabular component that has migrated medial to Kohler's line. Adequate preoperative planning can predict which patients are at risk for vascular injury prior to surgery and can allow appropriate preoperative vascular consolation. I obtain a preoperative arteriogram in patients who have greater than 50% of the acetabular component medial to Kohler's line on an anterior-posterior (AP) radiograph to determine the proximity of the iliac vessels in relation to the acetabular component and associated screws (Figure 25-1). I elect to have a vascular surgeon perform a retroperitoneal approach and gain control of the iliac vessels prior to removing the components if the vessels are compressed or in direct contact with the components.

The quadrant system described by Wasielewski is a very useful clinical tool to avoid vascular injury during surgery. This system is based upon 4 acetabular quadrants that are formed by drawing a line from the anterior superior iliac spine through the center of the acetabulum into the posterior fovea. A second line is then drawn perpendicular to the first line at the midpoint of the acetabulum (Figure 25-2). The posterior superior and posterior inferior quadrants are the safest quadrants to place acetabular screws and also contain the most robust bone for screw fixation. Screws placed aberrantly within the anterior superior quadrant result in a potential risk of damage to the external iliac artery and vein while screws placed within the anterior inferior quadrant risk damage to the obturator artery.

Figure 25-1. AP pelvic radiograph of a 58-year-old female with a pelvic discontinuity due to medial migration of her acetabular component. A retroperitoneal approach was performed at the time of revision surgery to gain control of the common iliac artery and vein.

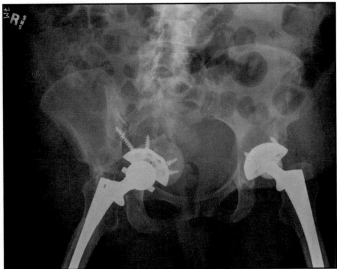

Figure 25-2. The quadrant system used to determine safe acetabular screw placement. Care must be taken if screws are placed in the anterior superior or anterior inferior quadrant to avoid injury to the external iliac vein and obturator artery, respectively.

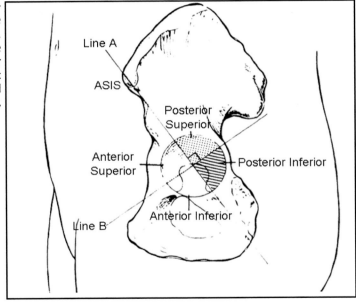

Vascular injuries are generally noticed immediately when they occur due to the profuse bleeding encountered within the acetabulum. Occasionally, the first clinical sign may be a drop in the patient's blood pressure or unexplained tachycardia. These phenomena can occur if a screw is placed into the acetabulum component following arterial damage. In this instance, the screw may prevent blood form extravasating into the acetabulum and result in bleeding that extends into the retroperitoneal space. If severe bleeding is encountered, the first step should be to pack the wound and attempt to provide compression at the site of injury. The anesthesiologist should be informed immediately and several units of compatible blood should be obtained along with a method of rapid infusion. The surgeon must then decide if the bleeding can be controlled with compression and if a major vessel has been damaged. Immediate vascular surgical consolation should be obtained if a direct injury is suspected and ongoing blood loss is occurring. Compression can continue to be used in an attempt to obtain hemostasis if the patient remains hemodynamically stable without the need for blood products or vasopressors. However, if the patient becomes hemodynamically unstable, the wound should be packed, the patient should be placed into a supine position, and a retroperitoneal approach performed to gain control of the bleeding. The retroperitoneal approach is performed by making a curvilinear incision slightly anterior to the anterior superior iliac spine to a point where the femoral pulse can be felt at the inguinal crease. The skin and fat are incised down to the level of the external oblique fascia. The external oblique, internal oblique, and transverses abdominus muscles are divided to reach the retroperitoneum. Blunt dissection is used to identify the external iliac artery and the more posterior external iliac vein. Vessel loops can be placed around these vascular structures to provide hemostasis until appropriate vascular surgical repair can occur.

A 45-Year-Old Patient With Hip Fusion Is Now Complaining of Increasing Back Pain. What Should I Do?

Steve Mussett, MD, FRCSC
Paul E. Beaulé, MD, FRCSC

Arthrodesis has historically been a reliable treatment option for a number of end-stage hip joint pathologies, providing effective symptom relief and allowing return to an active lifestyle. The long-term effects on the surrounding joints has, however, been well-documented and for this reason, together with improved total joint technique and bearing surfaces, we find a patient reluctance to accept fusion as a treatment option and furthermore, an increasing demand for conversion to total joint arthroplasty to alleviate symptoms and improve range of motion.

The common presenting complaints after a long-standing hip fusion are back pain (50% to 65%) frequently associated with degenerative radiographic findings. Knee pain is also a frequent finding both ipsilateral (30% to 76%) and contralateral (13% to 33%). Contralateral hip pain may also develop (13% to 32%) and this too usually occurs with advanced degenerative radiographic changes.

Bearing this in mind, the most common indications for conversion are disabling back pain (Figure 26-1), ipsilateral knee pain, and contralateral hip pain. Further indications include a malpositioned fusion with poor function, a symptomatic pseudoarthrosis, or the need to perform a knee replacement on the ipsilateral side. The last is associated with improved total knee functional outcomes after fusion take down as opposed to total knee replacement alone.

Confronted with this scenario, our first step is a thorough history, identifying patient symptoms, functional limitations, and desired level of activity. The key is to identify the source of the pain to ensure that a conversion will in fact improve the discomfort. Further information such as the original diagnosis, indication for fusion, surgical technique,

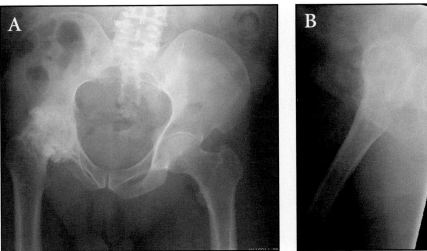

Figure 26-1. A 66-year-old patient with spontaneous hip fusion post sepsis as a young adolescent complaining of lower back pain.

instrumentation used, and associated complications form an integral part of the preoperative workup. Our examination focuses on inspection of the skin, previous incision sites, fusion position, and leg length measurements. A crucial exam finding is the state of the abductors. Absent or weak abductors are associated with poor functional outcomes and are considered by some to be a contraindication to take down. Computer tomography (CT) scan or magnetic resonance imaging (MRI) may be used to assess abductor status; however, we find inspection and palpation of the abductor mass for active contraction the most reliable means of assessment. The remainder of the exam includes examination of the surrounding joints as well as a thorough neurovascular assessment of both limbs.

Planning is completed with radiographs including an anterior-posterior (AP) pelvis and true lateral of the hip and femur as well as Judet views to assess acetabular bone stock. CT scan is useful to further delineate the distorted anatomy and assess bone stock. This allows us to identify potential problems with inadequate bone stock and abnormal anatomy as well as identify landmarks that may prove useful during take down. Templating the opposite side as a reference is recommended if it is anatomically normal.

Our incision and approach are based on previous incisions and fusion technique and fixation used. We prefer a lateral decubitus position with a posterolateral incision, which permits a trochanteric slide osteotomy, which may be required for acetabular exposure. A femoral neck osteotomy is made based on the preoperative template of the normal side. The lesser trochanter, pubofemoral arch, or screw holes can also be used as a guide to the osteotomy level. In addition, an intraoperative x-ray with the planned femoral neck cut marked with a K-wire can also be very useful. Acetabular preparation begins as templated relative to the femoral neck cut. The teardrop can be estimated by palpating the superior rim of the obturator foramen. The acetabulum is then reamed in standard fashion, paying attention to column and medial wall thickness. If at all concerned, intraoperative fluoroscopy is recommended to verify position. We prefer an uncemented cup with supplemental screw fixation if needed. The femur is prepared in standard fashion with insertion of either a cemented or uncemented stem. Careful attention should be paid

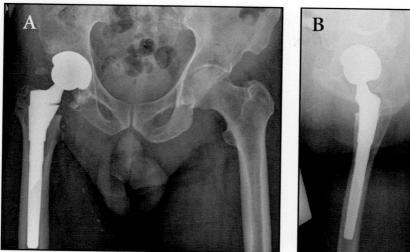

Figure 26-2. Twelve-month post-total hip replacement with (A) a modular stem and (B) a 36-mm head metal-on-metal bearing.

to leg length when trialing and we advise locating the sciatic nerve to assess its mobility with components in place. Because of the risk of hip instability, usage of a large femoral head may be advisable (Figure 26-2) and a constrained liner should be considered in case of absent abductors and an unstable trial.

On rare occasions, it is necessary to strip the abductors off the outer ileum to provide adequate length. Direct suture to the femur or suture of tensor fascia to the greater trochanter has also been described.

Successful take down usually improves pain, walking, and overall function with good patient satisfaction. Back pain is frequently relieved (73% to 92%) too as is ipsilateral knee pain and contralateral hip pain. Range of motion and leg length discrepancy are also significantly improved. Survivorship is comparable to primary joint replacement if multiple surgeries have not been performed and the patient is older than 50 years. Amongst others, the more frequent conversion complications include infection, dislocation, sciatic nerve injury, trochanteric detachment, and heterotopic ossification.

Albeit challenging surgery with increased risk of complications, if well planned and executed, take down surgery provides relief of symptoms with high patient satisfaction and favorable outcomes in most circumstances.

Bibliography

Beaulé PE, Matta JM, Mast JW. Hip arthrodesis: current indications and techniques. *J Am Acad Orthop Surg.* 2002;10:249-258.

Hamadouche M, Kerboull L, Meunier A, Courpied JP, Kerboull M. Total hip arthroplasty for the treatment of ankylosed hips: a five to twenty-one-year follow up. *J Bone Joint Surg Am.* 2001;83:992-998.

Hardinge K, Murphy JC, Frenyo S. Conversion of hip fusion to Charnley low-friction arthroplasty. *Clin Orthop.* 1986;211:173-179.

Panagiotopoulos KP, Robbins GM, Masri BA, Duncan CP. Conversion of hip arthrodesis to total hip arthroplasty. *AAOS Instr Course Lect.* 2001;50:297-305.

I Am Doing a Routine Total Hip Arthroplasty and I Am Unable to Obtain Hip Stability. What Should I Do?

Hari Parvataneni, MD
Harry E. Rubash, MD

With a combination of meticulous preoperative planning and a reproducible, consistent operative technique, we have found it very uncommon to have unexpected intraoperative instability. Preoperative planning (including physical examination, templating, and implant selection) and operative technique (including achieving and checking for appropriate leg length, soft tissue tension, and component position as well as provocative testing of range of motion and impingement) are, therefore, the most important factors in avoiding this problem. Despite our best efforts, however, we may occasionally face this scenario.

Acceptable stability will vary somewhat depending on surgical approach. Generally, it is absence of dislocation or impingement at or beyond specific extremity positions during intraoperative testing: 90 to 120 degrees of flexion, 45 to 60 degrees of internal rotation at 90 degrees of flexion, position of sleep (30 to 45 degrees of flexion and 30 degrees of adduction), and maximal extension and external rotation. If this is not achieved, there is no better time to solve the problem and it can usually be done with a few simple "tweaks" or changes.

The first and most important step is to critically analyze each step of the procedure (Table 27-1). In our experience, this will solve the problem in the majority of cases. Common errors in evaluating many of the intraoperative parameters include a change in pelvic position, inadequate exposure/visualization of the acetabulum and femur, and failure to identify and use appropriate anatomic landmarks. Major technical errors (eg, component malposition) will be detected this way and must be corrected. Simply increasing neck lengths or head sizes may improve stability without having to correct these major errors, but the hip reconstruction will be suboptimal and other problems may occur.

Table 27-1

Aspects of a Total Hip Replacement That Should Be Critically and Systematically Evaluated With Intraoperative Instability

Preoperative Planning and Templating

- Review your preoperative notes (these should be available in the operating room).
- Verify the accuracy of the radiographs and the magnification.
- Did you restore leg length, offset, and soft tissue tension on templating?
- Are you restoring or maintaining the center of rotation?
- Is there any radiographic predictor for instability?—high offset anatomy, varus neck-shaft angle, long neck length, mismatch between stem size and required neck length and lateralized hip center (large medial osteophyte or thick medial wall).
- Did you choose an appropriate femoral component?—neck-shaft angle, neck length, offset, head size, and skirted femoral heads.

Intraoperative

- Verify all trials and opened implants. Are these what you intended and do they match your preoperative planning?
- Verify anesthesia and level of muscle relaxation (for general anesthesia).
- Is your center of rotation appropriate? The transverse acetabular ligament is a key landmark for this.
- Verify acetabular component position using internal landmarks (pubis, ischium, ilium, and transverse acetabular ligament) and external references (positioning device). Confirm appropriate pelvic position on the table! Beware of osteophytes!
- Verify femoral neck cut, depth of implant, lateralization, and anteversion.
- Check combined anteversion (coplanar test).
- Double check leg lengths using the standard technique you normally use.
- Check soft tissue tension with the appropriate muscle relaxation (Shuck test, dropkick test, Ober test, etc).
- Perform provocative testing for range of motion and impingement.
- Obtain radiographs—many of the above factors can be verified on a single radiograph with appropriate projection.

Implant Design/Selection

It is critical to understand the unique design features of the implants you are using: availability of lipped or lateralized liners, head size options, implant offset, difference in neck lengths/offset between femoral sizes and head neck angles. This information should be correlated with the requirements of the particular patient during the preoperative planning phase. The majority of patients will fall within the normal design range. It is crucial to detect the outliers ahead of time and then solve these problems during the operation (Figure 27-1).

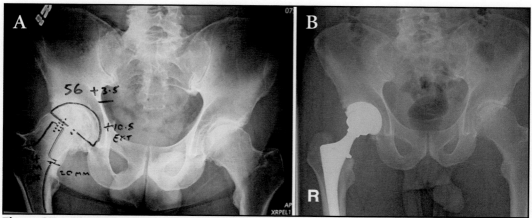

Figure 27-1. The importance of preoperative planning: (A) This patient has hips with high offset and long neck lengths. (B) To achieve stability, we used a high neck cut, high offset stem, a long neck length, and a lateralized liner. The hip was unstable without this combination, but this was known preoperatively.

Component Position

When assessing acetabular position, an osteophyte can be mistaken for the anterior or posterior walls and columns and can cause version errors. Forward or backward pelvic tilt can result in misjudged version, but intraoperative pelvic tilt (during manipulation) can influence cup inclination and this factor is often neglected. When assessing femoral version, it is important to not depend solely on proximal femoral landmarks (neck and intertrochanteric anatomy) as this can be misleading and some patients have abnormal proximal femoral version. Femoral anteversion should be correlated with the epicondylar axis of the knee with the knee flexed. Femoral anteversion may be altered before inserting the stem by altering the rasp position. Once correct, the actual implant can be inserted. Modular stems (with varying neck lengths, offset, and angles) allow varying of femoral version separate from the stem fixation position and may address this issue.

Impingement

Impingement should be detected during provocative testing. Osteophytes are major culprits and should be removed—do not forget femoral osteophyte! Trochanteric impingement on the pelvis (the pubis anteriorly and the ischium posteriorly) is under-recognized. This can be solved by improving trochanteric clearance (improving soft tissue tension) or by directly removing the impinging trochanter. An elevated rim liner is useful in many cases but can result in impingement in some instances and can be solved by using a standard liner or by placing the elevation in a different position. Longer necks are often skirted and impingement risk with skirted necks should be balanced with improved soft tissue tension.

Soft Tissue Tension

Instability will be solved in the majority of cases by restoring (or improving) soft tissue tension, achieving appropriate component position, and eliminating impingement. If more stability is required, adding a neck length, going to an extended offset neck, or going to a lateralized liner often improves the tension significantly. We will not hesitate to overlengthen a bit to achieve stability. We routinely counsel patients preoperatively about this and will reiterate this postoperatively if we do resort to that. Additionally, depending on the stem design, upsizing the stem may increase neck length without having to go to a skirted neck. Assessing soft tissue tension is subjective and needs to be standardized and consistent in terms of muscle relaxation, leg position, and testing. Measuring offset and lesser trochanter to center of neck distance before neck osteotomy and after reconstruction will prevent major discrepancies.

We do not use constrained liners in primary total hip arthroplasty and that option inherently places unacceptable forces on acetabular fixation. Stability and fixation are critical early goals, but it is conceivable that there will be the rare case requiring this option.

Conclusion

Unexpected instability should be rare and instability should be systematically and meticulously evaluated and solved immediately. It is tempting to rationalize and accept instability (especially milder degrees), but intraoperative instability equates to postoperative instability. We have never regretted spending a little extra time evaluating and fixing this problem right away.

Bibliography

Charles MN, Bourne RB, Davey JR, Greenwald AS, Morrey BF, Rorabeck CH. Soft-tissue balancing of the hip: the role of femoral offset. *Instr Course Lect.* 2005;54:131-141.

Della Valle AG, Padgett DE, Salvati EA. Preoperative planning for primary total hip arthroplasty. *J Am Acad Orthop Surg.* 2005;13(7):455-462.

Soong M, Rubash H, Macaulay W. Dislocation after total hip arthroplasty. *J Am Acad Orthop Surg.* 2004;12(5):314-321.

SECTION V

INTRAOPERATIVE ACETABULUM QUESTIONS

I Have a Portion of the Acetabular Component Uncovered During Acetabular Revision. Is This Is Okay, and How Much Uncoverage of the Component Is Acceptable to Use a Hemispherical Component Alone?

Michael O'Rourke, MD

I have found that using hemispherical trials in the desired implant location to judge adequate host-bone support is the most valuable tool for making decisions about how much uncoverage is acceptable.

During an acetabular revision hip arthroplasty, uncoverage of a portion of the acetabulum is a common occurrence. Cementless fixation has proven to be a successful and durable treatment for this scenario. Fixation of the acetabular component in both primary and revision settings is contingent on having a surface that allows ingrowth, minimizing micromotion below threshold to allow ingrowth, and obtaining intimate of this ingrowth surface to host bone.

For success, the minimum amount of bone contact necessary is essentially the amount that prevents micromotion below the threshold to allow ingrowth. The question of tolerable uncoverage has been controversial and confusing historically, partly related to limitations in quantifying the degree of uncoverage in retrospective studies. The majority of the literature regarding coverage of acetabular components and implant durability was based on judging uncoverage based on two-dimensional radiographic views. There are clearly limitations in resolving three-dimensional contact with two-dimensional radiographs. The controversy is further complicated by the mechanism of fixation. Many of the criteria for tolerable coverage and uncoverage relate to data with cemented acetabular cups and this probably has little applicability to cementless fixation. Theoretically, the durability of cementless fixation is better than cemented fixation due to adaptive responses in the bone supporting the implant at points of ingrowth.

There are many variables to consider when discussing host bone support of the cementless hemispherical cup. These include 1) percentage of the cup surface contacting host bone, 2) surface area of contact between the implant and host bone, 3) geometric location of the host-bone contact with the acetabular component (dispersion), 4) frictional coefficient of the ingrowth material, and 5) supplemental fixation (ie, screws). Figures of 50% to 60% host-bone coverage had been quoted as being necessary for durable fixation. It is generally believed that with increasing cup size, the percentage of cup contact to host bone may require a smaller percentage due to increasing overall surface area of contact. In addition, geometric location of host-bone contact with the cup is critically important. For example, if there is 50% "coverage" (contact with host bone) that supports the cup in a triangular fashion (like a tripod), the stability of the cup will be much greater than if that 50% is all in one hemisphere of the cup.

Using trials is a valuable tool in determining the net result of support to an implant and helping the surgeon determine overall if the supportive host bone is adequate for hemispherical fixation. I typically will use reamers to freshen margins of host bone and gauge the location of usable bone. Reaming during acetabular revision should be done cautiously to prevent removal of bone that otherwise may be supportive and necessary to achieve stable fixation. The size of the acetabular reamers may be increased to achieve greater bone contacting the spherical bone bed, being cognizant to avoid excessive bone removal in the anterior or posterior columns supporting the cup. After freshening the bone bed with a reamer, the trial implant (generally 1 mm greater than the last reamer placed) is inserted. It is important to place the cup in the desired cup position to gauge whether bone is supported in that location. The trial implant is evaluated for stability and those categories would include full inherent stability, partial inherent stability, and no inherent stability. Full inherent stability would be a trial that has a press-fit within the host bone and upon removal of the trial inserter, palpation of the rim of the trial implant around its circumference does not lead to migration or movement of that trial. Partial inherent stability would be a situation in which trial implant has some stability. After removal of the trial inserter, pressure placed on the rim of the trial implant leads to migration of the cup. Finally, no inherent stability would be a trial that does not gain any press-fit in the host bone. During the process of removing the trial inserter, the cup has migration.

In the setting of full inherent stability, hemispherical press-fit fixation without structural supplementation is generally acceptable and indicates adequate bone to allow bone ingrowth and durable fixation. In the setting of partial inherent stability, the decision would be made based on the location of the bone, whether increasing cup size would be desirable in order to achieve greater host-bone contact or in the setting where further reaming may compromise column support and/or lead to pelvic discontinuity, a decision is made regarding augmentation of the portion of the trial that is unsupported. This would be a scenario where structural bone allograft or other forms of structural augmentation such as modular acetabular revision components may be useful. Finally, the setting of no inherent stability would require either an increase in acetabular size to reach bone that is supportive and re-trialing and/or a determination that press-fit hemispherical fixation is not achievable, in which case either a nonhemispherical, modular augmentation technique, cemented fixation with use of a cage reinforcement, or custom implant should be utilized.

Use of screws in the primary setting is common, although press-fit fixation without screw fixation may be achievable with good long-term results. In the revision setting, with some degree of bone compromise and/or uncoverage, I choose to use screw fixation routinely. Screws are generally placed in locations where bone is present, being cognizant of locations with structures at risk. Posteroinferior and posterosuperior quadrants are safest. There are newer technologies that likely will change the stability of the initial fixation based on the porosity of implant material and frictional cofriction of these materials.

Conclusion

Many variables affect the durability and quality of initial fixation of hemispherical press-fit fixation in revision arthroplasty and I find it to be very useful to use the criteria of degree of inherent stability with trial implants to make the determination whether additional supplementation is necessary. I believe screw fixation is a useful augmentation in nearly all revision acetabular reconstructions and would generally place several screws where bone is available to gain purchase.

Bibliography

Hooten JP Jr, Engh CA Jr, Engh CA. Failure of structural acetabular allografts in cementless revision hip arthroplasty. *J Bone Joint Surg.* 1994;76B:419-422.

Paprosky WG, Perona PG, Lawrence JM. Acetabular defect classification and surgical reconstruction in revision arthroplasty: a 6-year follow-up evaluation. *J Arthroplasty.* 1994;9:33-44.

Shinar AA, Harris WH. Bulk structural autogenous grafts and allografts for reconstruction of the acetabulum in total hip arthroplasty: sixteen-year-average follow-up. *J Bone Joint Surg.* 1997;79A:159-168.

Templeton JE, Callaghan JJ, Goetz DD, et al. Revision of a cemented acetabular component to a cementless acetabular component: a ten to fourteen-year follow-up study. *J Bone Joint Surg.* 2001;83A:1706-1711.

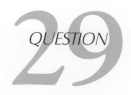
I Have a Patient With Severe Segmental Bone Loss in the Superior Dome of the Acetabulum. What Should I Do to Reconstruct This Defect?

Steven H. Weeden, MD
Steven Ogden, MD

Porous, noncemented acetabular implants in revision surgery have provided far superior results than cemented components and should be the method of choice for most acetabular revisions. However, a noncemented acetabular component relies upon biological fixation (ingrowth) to provide long-term stability. Revision of an acetabulum in the setting of severe segmental bone loss continues to provide a challenging problem. In Paprosky Type IIIA and IIIB acetabular defects, the remaining acetabular rim may not provide the support needed to maintain absolute component stability to allow for bone ingrowth.[1]

The exact amount of biological fixation needed to provide durable implant stability is unknown. Most surgeons would agree that 50% to 60% of implant to host bone contact is needed—as viewed in the coronal plane on an anteroposterior radiograph.[2]

In Paprosky Type I and II defects, the acetabular rim will usually support a hemispherical cup with less than 30% of the cup uncovered. This may allow for press-fit fixation alone. Nevertheless, screw supplementation should be considered whenever absolute stability cannot be achieved by the press-fit.

Micromotion between the implant and the host bone, as little as 40 to 50 μm, can lead to meager or no bone ingrowth and subsequent failure.[2] Added peripheral screw supplementation has provided durable acetabular implant fixation with excellent long-term results when less than 30% to 50% of the cup is uncovered.[3] In contrast, Paprosky Type III bone defects had a 19% failure rate when a hemispherical cup with peripheral screw augmentation was used.[3]

Figure 29-1. Preoperative radiograph of Paprosky Type III defect.

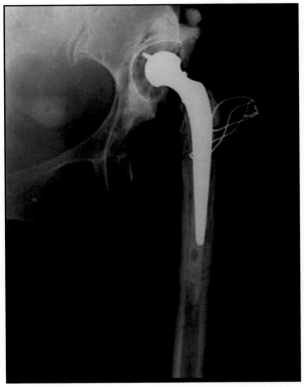

Several options have been studied to allay this complicated problem. Structural "number 7" allografts, antiprotrusio rings and cages with morcellized allograft, custom triflange components, and oblong cups have provided excellent short-term results but have led to loosening and failure at mid- to long-term follow-up.[4] Distal femoral or proximal femoral bulk allograft with a cage has been successfully used when the implant contacts less than 50% host bone.[5,6] However, this nonbiological fixation may lead to failure as the severity of the defect worsens with time.

In contrast, modular tantalum metal augments can be used to support a hemispherical shell when less than 50% of host bone is available for biological fixation. Tantalum augments are porous and have a low modulus of elasticity, providing an optimal environment for bone ingrowth. Short-term results have been very promising and the biological fixation achieved may lead to durable fixation in the long term.[5]

Preoperative Planning

Preoperative radiographs are studied for component migration. Superolateral or superomedial migration greater than 2 to 3 cm in reference to the superior obturator line with mild to moderate ischial lysis is consistent with Paprosky Type III acetabular defects (Figure 29-1). Computed tomography scans may be obtained to further identify bone loss and are needed if custom triflange components are to be utilized. Preoperative laboratory evaluation may include a C-reactive protein (CRP) and an erythrocyte sedimentation rate

(ESR) and are correlated with intraoperative frozen sections and cell counts to evaluate for the presence of infection.

Positioning of the patient is critical and the orientation of the pelvis relative to the floor must be known, as the normal landmarks are often distorted. A posterolateral approach is frequently used and can be made extensile by an extended trochanteric osteotomy.

If there is spherical bone remodeling, some Type 3 defects may be treated with jumbo shells with dome screw fixation. However, in revision cases with Type 2 or Type 3 defects, oblong remodeling can occur and hemispherical cups require structural allograft or trabecular metal augments superiorly. Moving the hip center superiorly and using a hemispherical cup is another option, but this is less desirable. Custom triflange implants may also be used and do provide biological fixation; however, they are expensive and require significant time to manufacture. Tantalum metal augments can be customized by reaming or with the use of a burr and are readily available. We currently prefer tantalum metal augments over the use of structural allograft.

Operative Technique

A posterolateral approach is frequently preferred with a posterior capsulotomy. If increased exposure is needed, a capsulectomy is performed. An extended trochanteric osteotomy will assist in the exposure of the acetabulum or removal of the femoral implant, if necessary.

The acetabulum is exposed in a subperiosteal fashion to include the posterior column and the ilium. Removal of the existing components are carried out and a systematic debridement of the acetabulum is undertaken to asses the remaining bone stock.

An attempt is made to identify the original hip center and limited reaming is carried out to achieve 2 points of contact, usually posteroinferiorly and anterosuperiorly. This allows for an intimate contact between the implant and host bone and may provide some inherent stability.

Tantalum metal augments can be added for additional fixation prior to or after the implant has been placed. A majority of the time the augment can be added after the cup has been placed and provisionally fixed with screws, usually on opposite sides of the implant.[5,6] The posterosuperior quadrant of the acetabulum is the safest for screw placement. The augment-cup interface is secured with polymethylmethacrylate and the augment is secured to the host bone with 6.5-mm cancellous screws (Figure 29-2). If the host bone or augment has a mismatch, either can be contoured using a burr to optimize the surface contact area to promote bone ingrowth.

Postoperatively, patients are instructed to partially weight bear on the operative leg with use of a walking aid for a minimum of 6 weeks. Patients must also utilize hip precautions with a hip abduction orthosis for 6 weeks due to the risk of dislocation associated with revision surgery.[5]

Figure 29-2. Postoperative radiograph at 1 year after hip revision with tantalum metal augment and screw fixation.

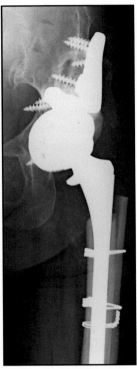

References

1. Paprosky WG, Perona PG, Lawrence JM. Acetabular defect classification and surgical reconstruction in revision arthroplasty: a 6-year follow-up evaluation. *J Arthroplasty.* 1994;9(1):33-44.
2. Sporer SM, Paprosky WG, O'Rourke M. Managing bone loss in acetabular revision. *J Bone Joint Surg Am.* 2005;87:1620-1630.
3. Weeden SH, Paprosky WG. Porous-ingrowth revision acetabular Implants secured with peripheral screws: a minimum twelve-year follow-up. *J Bone Joint Surg Am.* 2006;88:1266-1271.
4. Chen W, Engh CA, Hopper RH, Mcauley JP, Engh CA. Acetabular revision with use of a bilobed component inserted without cement in patients who have acetabular bone-stock deficiency. *J Bone Joint Surg Am.* 2000; 82:197-206.
5. Weeden SH, Schmidt RH. The use of trabecular metal implants for Paprosky 3a and 3b defects. Presented at: AAHKS Meeting; November 2006; Dallas, TX.
6. Weeden SH, Schmidt RH. The use of tantalum porous metal implants for Paprosky 3A and 3B defects. *J Arthroplasty.* 2007;22(6):151-155.

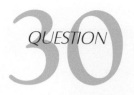
I Am Doing an Acetabular Revision While Retaining the Femoral Component and Cannot Get the Proximal Femur Out of the Way. What Should I Do?

Andrew H. Glassman, MD, MS

Your "next move" in this situation depends upon the initial approach utilized. During preoperative planning for an isolated cup revision, one should always select an approach that can be easily extended if the need arises. My preference in this situation is the posterolateral approach. It is appropriate for cup revision under the following circumstances:

* Simple revisions of cemented or cementless cups when structural allograft is not required.

* Conversions: Revisions of modular endoprosthetic or bipolar arthroplasties to fixed cups.

* Cup revision as above when there is osteolysis involving the greater trochanter and trochanteric healing after standard osteotomy is less predictable (Figure 30-1).

* No significant change in leg length is required (eg, 1 cm or less).

Difficulty with acetabular exposure when using the posterolateral approach is attributable to the inability to displace the proximal femur anteriorly. The major restraints to femoral displacement are the tendinous insertion of the gluteus maximus, the anterior capsule, and the direct head of the rectus femoris. The entire tendinous insertion of the gluteus maximus is released with cautery. Proceed medially, dividing just the tendinous fibers and leaving a cuff of about 1 cm on the femur for reattachment during closure. Deep to the tendon, the cautery is redirected anteriorly and the direct muscular attachments of

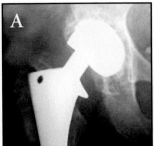 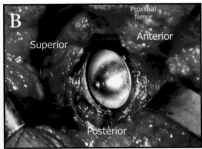 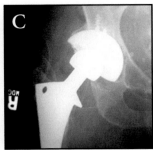

Figure 30-1. A failed cementless acetabular component in the presence of a well-fixed extensively porous-coated monoblock stem. There is extensive periacetabular and greater trochanteric osteolysis. (A) Preoperative anterior-posterior radiograph. (B) Acetabular exposure utilizing the posterior approach. (C) Postoperative radiograph.

the gluteus maximus and adductor magnus are stripped from the femur. The dissection is carried cephalad through the quadratus femoris until the entire lesser trochanter can be visualized. Complete anterior capsulotomy is recommended. This is best accomplished by retracting the femur laterally with a bone hook placed just distal to the lesser trochanter, internally rotating the femur, and placing a long Mayo scissor in the iliopsoas tendon sheath. The scissor is used to protect the tendon and femoral neurovascular structures by pulling the capsule posteriorly while dividing it between the scissor blades with cautery. A curved retractor is placed through the capsulotomy and over the anterior acetabular wall. The handle is then gently levered anteriorly and femur is internally rotated about 30 degrees. The direct insertion of the rectus femoris is then visualized and released from its insertion into the anterior inferior iliac spine and anterior superior rim of the acetabulum. This is greatly facilitated if the assistant simultaneously retracts the proximal femur anteriorly while progressively externally rotating the hip. If all of the above-described releases are adequate, the proximal femur will drop over the anterior rim of the pelvis, affording you excellent exposure of the anterior acetabulum (see Figure 30-1B).

Sometimes, it is easier and safer to proceed with a trochanteric osteotomy. My preference is the sliding trochanteric osteotomy. Its principal advantages in acetabular revision are improved exposure of the anterior and superior aspects of the acetabulum. The osteotomy is well suited for cases in which leg length must be altered more than 1 cm, and is resistant to proximal trochanteric "escape" if non-union occurs. The broader reattachment surface helps ensure bony union, even in the presence of trochanteric osteolysis. This approach should be considered for isolated acetabular revision when:

* Significant bone stock damage exists (noncontained rim defects) and structural allograft is required.
* A posterior column disruption requires plating.
* Trochanteric osteolysis exists.
* Significant (eg, greater than 1 cm) change in leg length is required.

The principal features of the sliding trochanteric osteotomy are the removal of a longer, thinner, and more vertical segment of the greater trochanter than that removed for traditional osteotomy, and the preservation of the vastus lateralis attachment to the distal aspect of the osteotomized segment (Figure 30-2). The 3 myofascial layers of the hip are

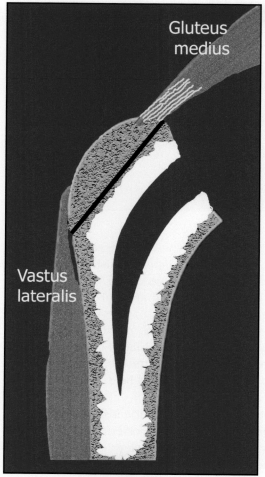

Figure 30-2. Schematic depiction of the sliding trochanteric osteotomy.

isolated and preserved during the dissection. The first layer is the fascia lata and the iliotibial band. The second is the gluteus medius and the vastus lateralis with the osteotomized segment of the greater trochanter between them. The third layer is composed of the gluteus minimus and the short external rotators.

Proximally, the tensor fascia lata must be thoroughly separated from the abductors. Placing the hip in a "figure of four" position (flexion, abduction, external rotation) facilitates this. The anterior border of the gluteus medius is identified and the interval between it and the gluteus minimus is defined. The interval between the gluteus medius and minimus is developed from posteriorly to anteriorly to complete the dissection begun anteriorly. Next, the fascia overlying the vastus lateralis is incised beginning at the vastus ridge proximally and extending distally just anterior to the intermuscular septum. Initially, the fascial division is carried out over a distance of 10 to 12 cm but can later be extended as far distally as circumstances require. The vastus lateralis muscle is elevated from the anterior and lateral aspects of the femoral shaft and held there with one or more Bennett retractors. The osteotomy begins just medial to the insertion of the gluteus medius into the greater trochanter, but lateral to the insertion of the gluteus minimus. Distally, it exits just beyond

Figure 30-3. Acetabular exposure with the sliding trochanteric osteotomy.

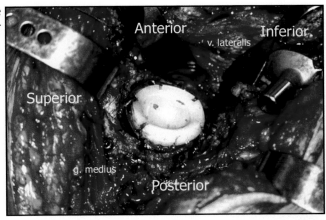

the vastus ridge. If these landmarks are used, the osteotomy will be longer (generally 5 to 6 cm), thinner (approximately 1.5 cm thick proximally and tapering distally), and more vertical than a traditional osteotomy. After completing the osteotomy, the trochanteric fragment remains tethered to the proximal femur by scar and anterior pseudocapsule. Extend the knee and gradually flex and externally rotate the hip. At the same time, retract the trochanteric fragment anteriorly and laterally and divide any capsule or scar tissue tethering it to the proximal femur. The intermediate myofascial layer, composed of the vastus lateralis distally, the gluteus medius proximally, and the thin segment of osteotomized trochanter between them, can now be "slid" anteriorly and held in place with the anterior jaw of a Charnley hip retractor.

The gluteus minimus attachment to the remaining trochanteric bed is divided and tagged. Next, the interval between the piriformis muscle and the posterior-inferior border of the gluteus minimus is scored with cautery and the minimus is elevated from the ilium sufficiently to expose the superior rim of the acetabulum. The hip is internally rotated and the short external rotators, from the piriformis down to and including the quadratus femoris, are stripped from the proximal femur. The hip is dislocated laterally by combining hip flexion, adduction, and external rotation. The leg is placed in a sterile bag affixed to the operating table anteriorly. Mobilization of the proximal femur may require partial or complete release of the iliopsoas tendon. During acetabular exposure, the proximal femur is retracted posteriorly and inferiorly with the posterior jaw of the Charnley retractor. Do this and you will have no trouble with acetabular exposure (Figure 30-3).

Closure is begun by suturing the gluteus minimus tendon to the undersurface of the gluteus medius at its insertion into the osteotomized trochanteric fragment using heavy, nonabsorbable suture. Two drill holes, each 2 mm in diameter, are drilled from posterior to anterior through the base of the lesser trochanter. Two 18-gauge cobalt chromium wires, each approximately 50 cm in length, are passed through these holes, leaving an equal amount anteriorly and posteriorly. Two sets of superior and inferior 2-mm holes (a total of 4 holes) are then drilled from lateral to medial through the trochanteric bed, one set anterior to the femoral prosthesis and one set posterior to it. The previously placed wires are then passed through these holes. Corresponding holes are then placed through the osteotomized segment of the greater trochanter and the wires are passed through them (Figure 30-4). The wires are then tightened over the lateral aspect of the trochan-

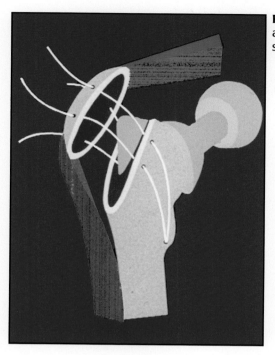

Figure 30-4. Recommended technique for re-attaching the greater trochanter following the sliding trochanteric osteotomy.

ter with an appropriate tightener. The vastus lateralis fascia is repaired with a running locking suture. Drains are placed within the joint. The tendons of the piriformis and the obturator internis are sutured through drill holes in the posterior aspect of the greater trochanter. The remaining closure is routine.

Bibliography

Glassman AH. Complications of trochanteric osteotomy. *Orthop Clin North Am.* 1992;23:321.

Glassman AH, Engh CA. The removal of porous-coated femoral hip stems. *Clin Orthop.* 1992;285:164.

Glassman AH, Engh CA, Bobyn JD. A technique of extensile exposure for total hip arthroplasty. *J Arthroplasty.* 1987;2:11.

I See a Fracture While Inserting an Acetabular Component With a 2-mm Press-Fit. The Component Is No Longer Stable. Now What Should I Do?

Todd Sekundiak, MD, FRCS

An iatrogenic fracture of the acetabulum can occur from 2 causes. The first is from transmitting reasonable force to compromised bone. The other is from placing excess force on bone that would not otherwise be compromised in a normal arthroplasty situation. Recognizing one's own ability to produce a fracture will allow the surgeon the ability to also avoid the fracture. A fracture of the acetabulum is only an error if unrecognized and if the cup is left unstable. Obviously, the more compromised the patient's bone stock, the more suspicious the surgeon must be.

It is the character of the fracture and the relevant stability of the implant that determines the management protocol. In general, the fracture patterns that can occur are the following: central "punch-out" lesions, rim or wall fractures, or transverse "discontinuity" fractures. When a fracture occurs, most situations can be managed by accepting the compromised stability and using a press-fit cup with screw augmentation. Do not be afraid to discard the component because it is of the wrong diameter or style to accommodate the created instability. The financial burden to the hospital or the patient will be far less by opening an additional component than an additional hospitalization to fix the failed arthroplasty.

Avoidance of fractures is one of the best initial treatments for acetabular fractures. With patients who are osteopenic, suspicion is prudent. Sometimes, it is difficult for me to judge how much osteopenia is present. In these situations, I use the acetabular reamer to initially remove the cartilage in the host acetabulum. Then, I place the reamer in reverse, and upsize my reamer till I get my adequate press-fit and a bleeding ingrowth surface. Reverse reaming is safe. It acts like an acetabular sound, allowing the surgeon to template the size of the acetabulum. This is similar to using acetabular trials but with the added advantage of mechanically débriding the acetabulum at the same time. All this can be done without concern for plunging through the subchondral plate of the acetabular floor and producing an unstable situation. If the bone is more sclerotic than initially anticipated, I simply return the reamer to the forward direction and stepwise ream to a larger diameter or more accommodating acetabular bed.

Another common error occurs when the surgeon feels the reamer needs to mimic the position of the acetabular component. Remember, the reamer is hemispherical so it can be placed in any direction and will still ream a hemisphere. With inspection and palpation, the surgeon should direct the reamer to remove the desired bone and cartilage to obtain an adequate press-fit. There is no need to mimic the position of the cup, which can inadvertently direct the reamer to remove a wall or column because of deforming soft tissues or femoral bone. In other words, push or pull the reamer handle to combat the deforming forces and ream the bone that is required.

Remember, the definition of 2-mm press-fit means different things depending on the morphology of the component. An eccentrically shaped or "dual-geometry" cup will fit differently than a hemispherical component. It is also important to understand the nomenclature of a cup. The cup may be described as a certain diameter, but with its dual geometry, the cup may actually be 2 mm larger than described at the rim. This produces a 4-mm fit rather than the expected 2-mm fit, if reamed to 2 mm smaller than the labeled diameter. The opposite issue occurs with components that are a partial hemisphere (165- or 170-degree) shape and will fit less aggressively than a full (180-degree) cup of the same described diameter. Further, a 2-mm press-fit in a smaller diameter cup creates more hoop stresses than a 2-mm press-fit in a larger diameter cup because of the relative difference in the ratios of the cup diameters. Finally, spikes, or an extremely roughened porous-ingrowth surface, may engage asymmetrically in the acetabulum prior to fully seating the component. Further impaction of the component produces asymmetric stresses on the acetabular wall and could possibly result in a fracture.

To avoid iatrogenically producing fractures, I avoid eccentrically or excessively reaming the acetabulum. With normal 2-mm press-fit, a cup is maintained in position by the acetabulum deforming in an elastic manner, and these hoop stresses are then used to maintain the position of the acetabular component. With excess or asymmetric reaming, the structural acetabular bone is lost and the acetabulum becomes more plastic. When attempting press-fit fixation, the normal "tight" fit is lost as the hoop stresses created with insertion of the cup produce plastic rather than elastic deformation. After assessing the instability in the component or trial, the surgeon may mistakenly "upsize" his or her component or "up ream" his or her acetabulum to improve his or her component stability. Toggling on the acetabular trial or component insertion handle will not produce the expected stability that one might normally expect. It is important to recognize the compromised bone has undergone plastic deformation, accept the compromised fixation, and augment the fixation with component screws. Further reaming or more aggressive press-fitting of the component usually will not lead to better fixation but more severe bone loss and a more complicated fracture pattern.

Reaming or impaction errors can produce an isolated or combination of fracture patterns. Reaming that weakens an isolated portion of the anterior, superior, or posterior

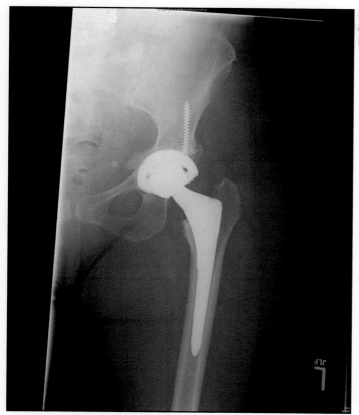

Figure 31-1. Central acetabular defect created by excess reaming the floor of the acetabulum.

portion of the wall can usually be ignored. A fracture of the acetabular wall of up to 30% of the acetabular surface can be easily accepted as long as the cup can be secondarily stabilized with adequate screw fixation. We know this can work as there is a great track record with porous cups in the revision setting where up to 30% of the acetabulum is not only fractured but missing. Stability must be unquestionable, however, once screw fixation is secured.

Excessive reaming that weakens or removes the floor of the acetabulum can also be managed similarly as long as there is enough rim of acetabulum to support the component. This is the one situation where we recommend judicious "over-reaming" of the acetabulum to gently expand the rim and allow a surface on the rim to rest the component on. This must be performed without further centralizing the reamers and removing more structural bone. I commonly employ the reverse reaming technique, previously described, to ensure adequate rim fit is obtained and seated medially enough to optimize fixation. This technique sounds the acetabulum to accept the oversized component without risking removal of more structural bone. If one does not "over-fit" these large central defects, the cup will migrate or swing into the defect, precluding stability and long-term fixation. The removed femoral head can be used as graft to augment fixation but should not be used to support the component (Figures 31-1 to 31-3).

Where reaming is not only eccentric but excessive, a combination of weakened regions occur that can produce a more significant fracture pattern. If continuity of the pelvis exists

Figure 31-2. Central acetabular defect created by excess reaming the floor of the acetabulum.

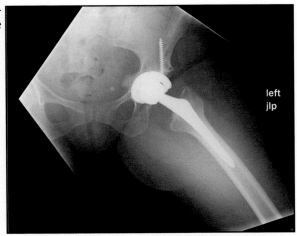

Figure 31-3. Long-term fixation maintained by screw fixation and rim fit of acetabular component. Medial grafting is used to augment ingrowth but not to support component.

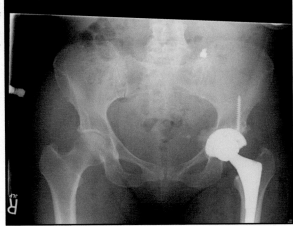

and enough surface area of the acetabulum remains, then a press-fit component with adequate and stable screw fixation can resolve the issue. Cup position and cup fixation should be directed in the posterior and superior direction. Because the cup is loaded in this direction, the surgeon wants to ensure the cup has the most intimate fit with the host bone in the remaining posterior superior acetabulum. This ensures the best potential for bone ingrowth and the best potential for long-term fixation. Initial screw fixation should also be directed in this manner to augment this intimate fit. Subsequent screws can be placed in any other direction to ensure stability but will then have less propensity to pull the cup away from the host-bone region of contact. We have not been successful in placing screws into the inferior hemipelvis but do attempt it if it can aid in stability.

For defects that are so large to preclude component stability, then the surgeon has no choice but to look at reconstruction cages or other constructs that provide an ilioischial bridge to prevent the cup from swinging and migrating out of position. The principles of cage fixation are beyond the scope of this question but should again be positioned in the posterior-superior direction of the acetabulum. The inferior extent of the cage is then impaled into the ischium to block medial and vertical migration of the acetabular component. Fixation onto the ischium can be performed but great caution and protection of the sciatic nerve must occur. Newer component augments or grafts may be needed for ancillary component fixation.

In general, when bone is of good quality, and a fracture occurs, I can usually maintain cup position with robust screw fixation that holds the cup till bone ingrowth can occur. Although rare, even when transverse fractures occur in this situation, acetabular component screw fixation can be used to secure the component. There are, however, caveats to this situation. First, the component should not be splaying the fracture fragments apart. This may require downsizing the component. Next, there must be adequate viable host bone to obtain ingrowth and late stability. Third, screw fixation superiorly must be robust and rigid. If possible, fixation inferiorly is also helpful. Finally, if in doubt, plate the posterior column to bridge the defect first and then follow the same preceding caveats. These transverse fractures occur acutely and have a better propensity to heal than those that occur in the revision setting.

A pelvic discontinuity that is seen from failed components and from associated osteolysis behaves differently than the above-described transverse fracture. A pelvic discontinuity in the revision setting is a pathologic fracture usually occurring from a chronic indolent process. Because of the atrophic nature of the fracture, they have much less propensity to heal. Although I attempt to stabilize and heal the discontinuity, this is less likely. Component stability and long-term fixation are usually achieved by stabilizing the component in a similar manner to the posterior-superior portion of the acetabulum as described in the previous paragraph. This might be the best that one can hope for in a severe defect, realizing that a source of chronic pain can result from the nonunion of the transverse acetabular fracture.

Avoid acetabular fractures with press-fit components at all costs. Understanding your patient's bone morphology and the behavior of the component and the instruments to insert it are the best ways to achieve that goal. When fractures occur, be prepared to "shift gears" by obtaining stability, not with the press-fit but with screw fixation. When fractures finally compromise stability of the hemipelvis, not only does the surgeon need to obtain stability of the component but also stability of the hemipelvis.

Bibliography

Berry DJ, Lewallen DG, Hanssen AD, Cabanela ME. Pelvic discontinuity in revision total hip arthroplasty. *J Bone Joint Surg Am.* 1999;81(12):1692-1702.

Haidukewych GJ, Jacofsky DJ, Hanssen AD, Lewallen DG. Intraoperative fractures of the acetabulum during primary total hip arthroplasty. *J Bone Joint Surg Am.* 2006;88(9):1952-1956.

Helfet DL, Ali A. Periprosthetic fractures of the acetabulum. *Instr Course Lect.* 2004;53:93-98.

Springer BD, Berry DJ, Cabanela ME, Hanssen AD, Lewallen DG. Early postoperative transverse pelvic fracture: a new complication related to revision arthroplasty with an uncemented cup. *J Bone Joint Surg Am.* 2005; 87(12):2626-2631.

While Reaming the Acetabulum, I Inadvertently Reamed Through the Medial Wall. What Should I Do?

William A. Lighthart, MD

Protrusion through the medial wall of the acetabulum during total hip arthroplasty can have several etiologies. It can be inadvertent, as in the case of overzealous medialization while reaming. It can be expected or even intentional during the reconstruction of a deficient acetabulum in developmental dysplasia of the hip (DDH). It can be unavoidable in cases of bone loss due to either osteolysis or component removal during revision surgery. Finally, it can be the result of pre-existing acetabular protrusio that is either a primary idiopathic condition or a secondary condition associated with inflammatory arthropathies, metabolic bone disorders, and several other causes.

The overall goal of any acetabular reconstruction is to achieve both initial inherent stability and long-term rigid fixation of the cup with recreation of the appropriate hip center of rotation of the hip. Excluding cases, such as postradiation necrosis, of host bone that is biologically compromised, my preferred method of reconstruction is with a cementless hemispherical cup.

As with any acetabular deficiency, I use the Paprosky classification system to characterize the severity of bone loss and help determine the potential to obtain fixation. The key to achieving both immediate and long-term fixation is the ability of remaining host bone to provide initial stability until ingrowth occurs. The amount of intact rim and therefore peripheral rim fit achieved by the implant along with the amount of coverage by host bone determines the overall stability and ingrowth potential. Using this system, violation of the medial wall would be classified as a Type IIC defect. Type IIC defects have less than 2 cm of superior migration of the hip center with a fully intact rim, >60% host-bone stock, intact columns, and full inherent stability of a trial implant.

Our preferred treatment for this type of defect is a hemispherical cementless cup with or without medial cancellous bone graft. Graft may be placed medially in order to reconstitute bone stock and fill contained defects. In the case of a primary total hip, autograft from the resected femoral head may be used and then impacted and shaped with an acetabular reamer in reverse. In revision settings, allograft is typically used. In either case, the graft is not structural and therefore not used to support the cup. Rim fit is used to support the cup and an intraoperative assessment of rim fit is obtained with trials. We routinely augment initial fixation of our cups in both primary and revision cases with screws.

Creation of a small inadvertent penetration of the medial wall during primary arthroplasty in a patient with normal bone does not routinely require bone graft. We would choose to use graft in cases where reconstitution of bone stock was deemed necessary. This could include revision surgery where defects encountered may be some combination of contained and uncontained. A large violation of the medial wall in a relatively young patient may result in lack of bone stock for future potential revision surgery. This may also be a situation in which bone grafting is warranted. Finally, cases of pre-existing protrusio, whether idiopathic or secondary to a known etiology, warrant special consideration.

Acetabular protrusio is a condition wherein the femoral head migrates medially and superiorly, violating Kohler's line. This migration of the head creates an oblong shape to the acetabulum with a medial wall that may be either thin and nonsupportive or violated primarily. Many different techniques for the reconstruction of this condition have been described. Our preference is to ignore the depth of the socket and ream the viable bone at the periphery of the acetabulum in order to achieve a rim fit. As in other cases, if adequate initial stability with at least 60% coverage of the cup by host bone can be achieved, an excellent chance of ingrowth and long-term stability may be expected. We would then fill the medial depth of the oblong acetabulum with particulate graft in order to recreate a hemispherical shape and reconstitute bone stock.

Regardless of the cause of medial wall violation, if adequate rim fit and implant coverage may not be obtained with a hemispherical porous cup alone, then another method of reconstruction should be chosen.

Bibliography

Della Valle CJ, Berger RA, Rosenberg AG, Galante JO. Cementless acetabular reconstruction in revision total hip arthroplasty. *Clin Orthop Relat Res.* 2004;420:96-100.

Harris WH. Management of the deficient acetabulum using cementless fixation without bone grafting. *Orthop Clin North Am.* 1993;24(4):663-665.

Heekin RD, Engh CA, Vinh T. Morcellized allograft in acetabular reconstruction: a post-mortem retrieval analysis. *Clin Orthop.* 1995;319:184-190.

Paprosky WG, Perona PG, Lawrence JM. Acetabular defect classification and surgical reconstruction in revision arthroplasty: a 6-year follow-up evaluation. *J Arthroplasty.* 1994;9(1):33-44.

SECTION VI

INTRAOPERATIVE
FEMUR QUESTIONS

I WAS IMPACTING A TAPERED FEMORAL COMPONENT AND I SEE A SMALL CRACK OF THE CALCAR. WHAT SHOULD I DO?

Michael E. Berend, MD

Uncemented stem utilization has increased over the past decade. With its rise in popularity so have proximal cracks in the femoral calcar.[1,2] This has been reported not only with tapered components but with cylindrical stems as well.[3] The risk factors have been well studied[1,2,4] and include uncemented stems, female gender, anterior surgical approach, and a diagnosis leading to total hip replacement (THR) other than osteoarthritis. Combining an understanding of these risk factors with preoperative templating may help identify patients at risk for proximal femoral fracture and an alternative stem with reduced proximal geometry may be selected.[1]

If the crack in the calcar is identified either during broaching or final stem implantation, we have found excellent healing and stem stability with treatment with cerclage wiring techniques.[1] I have found it less expensive to use looped Luque wires than braided cables with similar clinical performance.[5]

The technique of cerclage wiring of a proximal femoral crack initially involves removal of the broach or stem followed by wire placement and reinsertion of the implant. I place the wire in the subperiosteal location above the level of the lesser trochanter. I tighten the wire prior to stem insertion. One can place morcellized cancellous autograft from the host acetabular reamings in the area of the fracture prior to closure. I place the wires above the level of the lesser trochanter in order to create a stable construct for hoop stress distribution during stem insertion. This has been studied in the laboratory and is an effective way to reduce fracture propagation and promote torsional stability.[6]

Early reports with patch-coated implants in a canine model demonstrated reduced ingrowth in the presence of a proximal fracture.[7] These authors recommended considering cemented stem insertion if a proximal femoral fracture was encountered intraoperatively. We have found that uncemented stem survivorship is superior to cemented stem survivorship if a proximal femoral fracture is encountered in long-term follow-up of both types of stem fixation[1] (Figure 33-1).

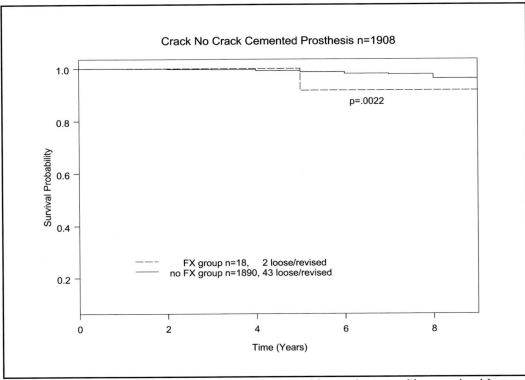

Figure 33-1. Kaplan-Meier survival analysis of cemented femoral stems with a proximal femoral fracture treated with cerclage wiring. (Reprinted from *J Arthroplasty,* Berend ME, Smith A, Meding JB, et al, Long-term outcome and risk factors of proximal femoral fracture in uncemented and cemented total hip arthroplasty in 2551 hips, 53, © 2006, with permission from Elsevier.)

If stem stability cannot be achieved with cerclage and a tapered stem then another treatment option is to proceed with distal fixation through a longer stem (Figure 33-2). This is not usually required in our experience unless the fracture proceeds well below the level of the lesser trochanter and has significant displacement.

Subsidence

My postoperative protocol has varied over time and for each surgeon within my group for cemented and uncemented stems. In patients with uncemented stems without a fracture, I routinely allow full weight bearing as tolerated and rapid weaning from a walker to a cane and then to no assist device as ambulatory strength returns. Most patients are using a cane or no assist device by 6 to 8 weeks with reduced incision protocols. In the presence of a proximal femoral fracture in which torsional stability has been achieved, I would recommend advancement of weight bearing as tolerated and use of a walker for 8 weeks. Berend et al[2] reported excellent stem stability, survivorship, and fracture healing when full weight bearing was allowed in hips receiving the Mallory-Head Porous stem (Biomet, Inc, Warsaw, IN) in which proximal femoral fractures were treated with cerclage wiring.

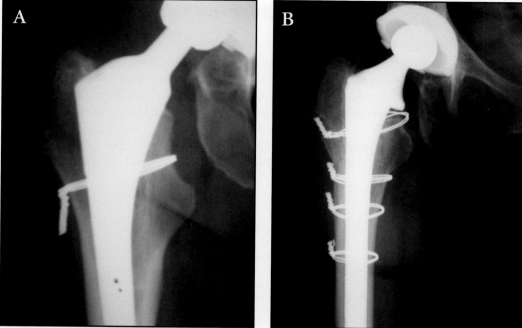

Figure 33-2. (A) Cerclage wiring with looped Luque wires above the level of the lesser trochanter resulting in stem stability with circumferentially coated, plasma-sprayed tapered titanium stem (BiMetric, Biomet Inc). (B) Long stem with diaphyseal fixation after a proximal femoral fracture in a revision setting with excellent stem stability.

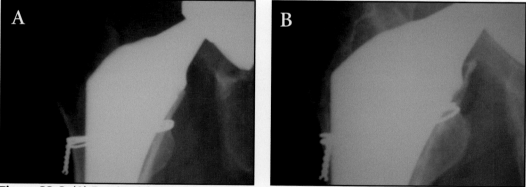

Figure 33-3. (A) Proximal femoral fracture encountered during implantation of an early uncemented stem design treated with cerclage wiring. (B) Subsidence occurred as the stem loosened requiring revision total hip arthroplasty.

With tapered stems in which a proximal femoral fracture was observed and treated with cerclage wiring regardless of weight bearing, I did not find significant evidence of subsidence.[1] Subsidence was found only as a sequelae of loosening in cemented and uncemented stems (Figure 33-3).

Conclusion

Proximal femoral fractures are encountered in approximately 4% of hips during tapered stem insertion.[1,2] Minimal changes in weight bearing are required. Patients at risk are those undergoing total hip arthroplasty for diagnoses other than osteoarthritis that may have altered proximal femoral metaphyseal geometry combined with anterior approach to the hip and female gender. Treatment with cerclage wiring above the level of the lesser trochanter with wires or cables has been shown to produce excellent survivorship with many different stem designs.[1,2] Patients and surgeons alike can be confident that intraoperative recognition and treatment of calcar cracks yields excellent long-term stem survivorship.

References

1. Berend ME, Smith A, Meding JB, et al. Long-term outcome and risk factors of proximal femoral fracture in uncemented and cemented total hip arthroplasty in 2551 hips. *J Arthroplasty*. 2006;21:53.
2. Berend KR, Lombardi AV, Mallory TH, et al. Cerclage wires or cables for the management of intraoperative fracture associated with a cementless, tapered femoral prosthesis: results at 2 to 16 years. *J Arthroplasty*. 2004; 19:17.
3. Schwartz Jr JT, Mayer JG, Engh CA. Femoral fracture during non-cemented total hip arthroplasty. *J Bone Joint Surg [Am]*. 1989;71:1135.
4. Moroni A, Faldini C, Piras F, et al. Risk factors for intraoperative femoral fractures during total hip replacement. *Ann Chir Gynaecol*. 2000;89:113.
5. Ritter MA, Lutgring JD, Davis KE, et al. A clinical, radiographic, and cost comparison of cerclage techniques: wires vs. cables. *J Arthroplasty*. 2006;21:1064.
6. Incavo SJ, DiFazio F, Wilder D, et al. Longitudinal crack propagation in bone around femoral prosthesis. *Clin Orthop Rel Res*. 1991;272:175.
7. Schutzer SF, Grady-Benson J, Jasty M, et al. Influence of intraoperative femoral fractures and cerclage wiring on bone ingrowth into canine porous-coated femoral components. *J Arthroplasty*. 1995;10:823.

Financial Disclosure: Dr. Berend is a consultant, receives royalties and research support from Biomet, Inc. He also receives research support from OREF, St. Francis Hospital, Zimmer, MCS, Inc.

I HAVE A PATIENT WITH SEVERE OSTEOLYSIS SURROUNDING HER GREATER TROCHANTER DURING A ROUTINE POLYETHYLENE LINER EXCHANGE. DO I NEED TO DO ANYTHING TO THIS AREA OF BONE LOSS AT THE TIME OF SURGERY?

William G. Hamilton, MD

The management of osteolysis in the greater trochanter remains a controversial and challenging problem in revision hip surgery. The indications for operative intervention have not been clearly defined, and the surgical techniques for bone grafting defects and fixation of trochanteric fractures have varied. Therefore, the decision-making process in this clinical scenario is difficult.

If greater trochanteric osteolysis is noted at the time of a routine polyethylene liner exchange, we routinely graft these lesions to slow the development of osteolysis and protect patients from future fractures. Technical pearls include the following:

* The cortical shell of the greater trochanter is usually very thin, and extreme care must be taken to avoid fracturing the bone.

* Carefully curette all fibrous debris out of the lytic lesion (Figure 34-1).

* Pulse lavage the region prior to placing any bone graft.

* Pack small morcellized allograft chips into the defect and consider mixing with a commercially available demineralized bone matrix to give the mixture viscosity and prevent migration of the graft.

Figure 34-1. Greater trochanteric osteolytic lesion adjacent to an extensively coated femoral stem. The lesion has been curettaged of all fibrous debris and lavaged to create a bleeding bone bed for subsequent grafting.

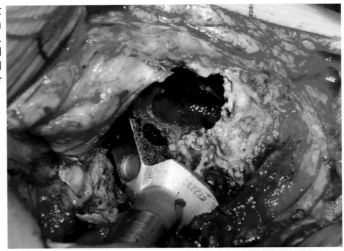

Figure 34-2. The same osteolytic lesion after packing with morcellized allograft.

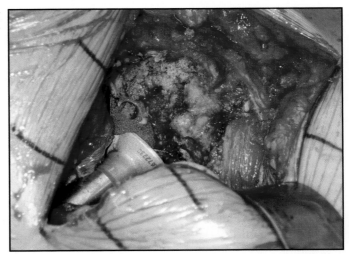

* Place graft material into the lesion and gently tamp it into place (Figure 34-2). Forceful packing can cause a fracture of the surrounding bone and should be avoided. The lesion is filled but care is taken to not leave any loose bone graft that could potentially migrate into the articular surface and cause third-body wear.

* After grafting the lesion, place a trial ball, reduce the hip, and take the hip through a full range of motion. Redislocate the hip and examine the graft to determine if any of the bone has dislodged. This graft can then be impacted or removed to prevent third-body wear from occurring.

* Lastly, if exposure and grafting of the lesion will compromise the integrity of the trochanter, then an isolated polyethylene exchange without bone grafting is performed. The polyethylene exchange alone will likely slow, if not halt, the progression of osteolysis in the trochanter.

Fixation of Greater Trochanteric Fractures

Several techniques of fixation have been described for fractures through osteolytic lesions in the greater trochanter. At our institution, we have seen few indications for trochanteric fixation, given that most fragments are small and heal with conservative management.[1] When fractures do occur at the time of surgery and the fragment is large enough to fix, several techniques have been employed.

My preference has been to use cerclage cables looped under the lesser trochanter and deep to the gluteus medius tendon in combination with grafting of the lytic defect. A transverse cable can be added for fractures that extend to the level of the lesser trochanter. If the fracture consists of several small bony fragments, I usually do not place any hardware; rather, I leave the soft tissue sleeve intact and allow fibrous consolidation postoperatively.

For larger fragments, trochanteric claws can be added and may improve fixation. However, they often lead to lateral trochanteric pain, and, therefore, all patients are told that the hardware will likely need to be removed at a separate operation once the bone has healed. Trochanteric plates that extend down the femoral shaft can be used in association with more distal femoral involvement such as an extended osteotomy with a trochanteric fracture or subtrochanteric involvement. However, this usually requires significant soft tissue stripping of the lateral femoral cortex and, therefore, is not routinely used.

Other fixation techniques of greater trochanteric fractures associated with osteolytic lesions have been described. Wang et al used a fixation technique with stainless steel wire in a figure-of-eight fashion.[2] The wire is passed through drill holes made distal to the vastus lateralis ridge and then looped around the abductor in a figure-of-eight fashion. The fracture can be bone grafted and then reduced with a towel clip. For lesions that involve the lesser trochanter or for larger fragments, additional fixation with an oblique wire can be added by looping the wire underneath the lesser trochanter. Treating fractures in this fashion, the authors describe good success, with 18 of 19 fractures healing at an average duration of a 3.8-year follow-up.

The use of a trochanteric claw plate to reattach the greater trochanter was described in 72 consecutive procedures.[3] Placement of the plate required detaching a portion of the vastus lateralis from the vastus ridge. Of the 72 hips treated with this claw plate, 51 patients went on to osseous union. Twelve patients failed and 9 had fibrous consolidation. Three of these plates required removal because of pain or implant breakage. Whiteside described a technique utilizing cerclage cables passed deep to the medius tendon and secured distally by a circumferential cable passed distal to the lesser trochanter.[4] This allows fixation of comminuted fractures and does not disrupt the blood supply. In addition, it does not leave exposed hardware that can cause pain and require later removal.

Postoperative Management

Patients treated for trochanteric fractures are routinely managed in an abduction orthosis. Motion is fixed at 30 degrees of abduction, allowing 0 to 90 degrees of hip flexion. Patients are allowed toe-touch weight bearing for a minimum of 6 weeks but can be extended to 12 weeks depending on the fracture type and fixation achieved. Therapists are instructed to avoid active abduction exercises during this period. We then advance to partial weight bearing using crutches or a cane until radiographic evidence of fracture healing is observed.

Results

At our institution, radiographs of 208 consecutive total hip arthroplasties performed with an extensively coated device and a mean follow-up of 12.2 years were examined.[1] The overall incidence of greater trochanteric osteolysis in these 208 patients was 19%. Of the 39 hips where osteolysis was noted in the greater trochanter, 9 (23%) sustained a fracture through the osteolytic lesion. Of the 9 patients identified with trochanteric fractures, 2 patients were asymptomatic and did not require immediate treatment. Four of the patients were treated with crutches and limited weight bearing for 6 weeks and went on to heal. Four patients ultimately underwent surgical intervention but not specifically for treatment of the fracture. One lesion was grafted due to its large size and underwent healing, and ultimately the lesion decreased in size. Despite the increase in size in some of the lesions, none went on to additional fractures after the index fracture had healed. If surgery with a concomitant polyethylene exchange was performed, the lesions tended to stabilize or decrease in size.

Conclusion

Treatment of osteolysis of the greater trochanter remains controversial. Fractures of the greater trochanter through osteolytic lesions, while often nondisplaced and easily treated with conservative management, can become technically very challenging if open reduction is required. Unless the fragment is large, we routinely allow these fractures to heal with a period of protected weight bearing and then only intervene surgically if they meet the criteria for the surgical management of osteolysis. Polyethylene exchange, debridement of the greater trochanteric region, and bone grafting are commonly performed at surgery. Thankfully, large displaced fractures of the greater trochanter are uncommon, and their treatment is a great technical challenge in revision hip surgery.

References

1. Claus AM, Hopper RH Jr, Engh CA. Fractures of the greater trochanter induced by osteolysis with the anatomic medullary locking prosthesis. *J Arthroplasty.* 2002;17(7):706-712.
2. Wang JW, Chen LK, Chen CE. Surgical treatment of fractures of the greater trochanter associated with osteolytic lesions. *J Bone Joint Surg A.* 2005;87-A:2724-2728.
3. Hamadouche M, Zniber B, Dumaine V, Kerboull M, Courpied JP. Re-attachment of the ununited greater trochanter following total hip arthroplasty: use of a trochanteric claw plate. *J Bone Joint Surg A.* 2003;85(7):1330-1337.
4. Whiteside LA. Trochanteric repair and reconstruction and revision total hip arthroplasty. *J Arthroplasty.* 2006; 21(4 supp):105-106.

Financial Disclosure: The author is a consultant, member of speakers bureau, and has received grant support from Depuy Orthopaedics in the past 12 months.

I Have a Patient With Severe Proximal Bone Loss That I Was Treating With an Extensively Coated Implant. During Insertion I Heard a Crack. What Should I Do?

R. Michael Meneghini, MD
Jeffrey L. Pierson, MD

Revision total hip arthroplasty in the setting of proximal femoral bone loss can be a challenging treatment problem. The majority of femoral revisions in this setting can be successfully treated with a cementless fully porous-coated femoral component of sufficient length to bypass the deficient proximal bone (exceptions may exist with femoral canals of large diameter and bone of extremely poor quality).[1] When bypassing the deficient bone, it has been recommended to obtain a minimum of 5 cm of intimate diaphyseal contact ("scratch fit") in order to obtain sufficient mechanical stability for clinical success.[2] Due to the frequently encountered scenario of poor bone quality and the need for an intimate diaphyseal "scratch fit" for adequate implant stability, there is a relatively high incidence of intraoperative fracture during insertion of cementless fully porous-coated implants and has a reported incidence of 0% to 20%.[2-5]

Prevention

As with the majority of intraoperative complications during revision hip arthroplasty, careful surgical technique and detailed preoperative planning can help minimize the incidence of femoral fracture during insertion of a fully porous-coated stem. Preoperative lateral radiographs must be reviewed with available femoral component templates to assess the degree and curvature of the femoral bow. In some instances, a bowed fully porous component may be required to prevent iatrogenic perforation or inadvertent femoral fracture. Adequate exposure must be obtained, and frequently an extended femoral osteotomy is required to remove the existing femoral component and adequately visualize the entrance of the intact diaphysis. If a femoral osteotomy is performed, it is suggested to minimize abrupt and sharp corners of the distal limb of the osteotomy to prevent a stress-riser that may propagate into a fracture with hoop stresses during component insertion. This can be achieved by using a pencil-tipped burr to create rounded osteotomy corners. Placing a prophylactic cerclage cable or double Luque wire distal to the osteotomy will also minimize diaphyseal hoop stresses, help prevent intraoperative fractures during implant insertion, and is recommended in all such cases.

The final implant should be measured with a hole-gauge to accurately measure the stem diameter, which can exhibit a degree of variability inherent in the manufacturing process. The canal is typically under-reamed by 0.5 mm for a straight stem and if the hole-gauge indicates a greater degree of interference fit, the canal should be reamed "line to line" prior to implant insertion. If a bowed femoral component is utilized, the surgeon should be prepared to over-ream the canal up 1 to 2 mm to allow for the subtle mismatch between the femoral canal and implant geometries.

Finally, during component insertion, the femoral component should be able to be inserted by hand to approximately 5 to 7 cm proud of its final position. If the interference fit is too great, the component should be removed and canal reamed up 0.5 mm larger. The prosthesis should advance gradually (approximately 1 mm) with each mallet blow and should be observed closely for any unexpected change in progressive seating until final seating.

If a "Crack" Is Heard or the Implant Suddenly Progresses Easily

If an audible or palpable "crack" is heard or felt, a femoral diaphyseal fracture is nearly certain. In addition, if any sudden increase in progressive seating is observed during stem insertion, intraoperative radiographs should immediately be obtained and a thorough inspection performed for a fracture. It is mandatory in this situation to obtain both anterior-posterior (AP) and lateral views, orthogonal to each other, to ensure complete visualization of the femoral cortex. It is helpful to have the preoperative radiographs available for comparison, as the nutrient artery can infrequently be interpreted as a nondisplaced fracture located obliquely along the posterior cortex of the femoral diaphysis. It is important if any suspicion of fracture is equivocal by intraoperative radiographs, additional views or direct visualization via extensile surgical exposure is required. Many surgeons recommend intraoperative radiographs regardless of clinical suspicion.[5]

Treatment

If a radiolucency is seen and consistent with an incomplete, nondisplaced fracture on direct visualization and if the adequate implant stability is present, it is recommended

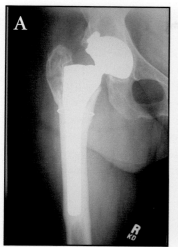
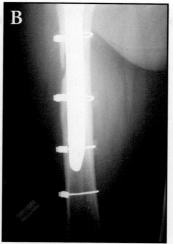
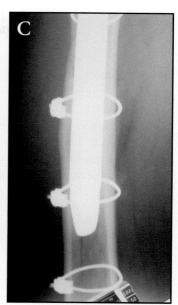

Figure 35-1. (A) Preoperative AP radiograph of a patient with a loose cementless femoral component. (B) Postoperative AP and (C) lateral distal femoral radiographs of the patient in Figure A at 6 months postoperatively demonstrating a healing nondisplaced fracture that occurred intraoperatively with insertion of a fully porous-coated stem. The cementless stem demonstrated adequate stability and a cerclage cable was placed past the distal extent of the fracture.

that cerclage cables or wires be placed to maintain fracture reduction and prevent propagation, ensuring that a wire is placed well past the most distal extent of the fracture (Figure 35-1). In most cases of proximal bone loss, if a fracture occurs, it frequently traverses distally to a point where bypassing the fracture with a longer prosthesis may not be possible. Therefore, if the femoral component is stable and the fracture is displaced, fracture reduction should be obtained in a manner consistent with accepted treatment of postoperative periprosthetic fractures around a well-fixed stem.[6] This should include allograft struts with or without a side-plate for biplanar stabilization, secured with cerclage cables or wires. The emergence of locking plate fixation may obviate the need for biplanar stabilization and has the benefit of preserving the osseous blood supply through the avoidance of the soft-tissue stripping that is required to place an allograft strut.

If rotational and axial stability are not present, the implant should be carefully removed and the fracture assessed by direct visualization. Fracture reduction is obtained and in many cases, it is preferable to insert a fluted, tapered, titanium (Wagner-type) modular prosthesis if subsequent implant stability is tenuous.[7] Additionally, these fractures should be supplemented with cancellous allograft or autograft bone when possible to facilitate union. Postoperatively, restricted weight bearing from 6 weeks to 3 months is recommended, depending on the extent of the fracture and the quality of implant stability and fracture fixation.

Outcomes

In their review of 8 intraoperative fractures that occurred while inserting a fully porous-coated femoral component, Chappell et al reported successful fracture union in 6 of 8 patients.[5] Treatment consisted of bicortical strut grafts and cables with restricted weight bearing. In a series of acute Vancouver B3 periprosthetic femur fractures (3 of which occurred intraoperatively during revision of a loose femoral component) treated with a fluted, tapered, titanium modular stem, Berry reported that all implants were stable and fractures healed at final follow-up.[7] If fracture healing is obtained and adequate implant stability preserved, these difficult intraoperative problems can be treated successfully.

References

1. Weeden SH, Paprosky WG. Minimal 11-year follow-up of extensively porous-coated stems in femoral revision total hip arthroplasty. *J Arthroplasty*. 2002;17(4 Suppl 1):134-137.
2. Paprosky WG, Greidanus NV, Antoniou J. Minimum 10-year-results of extensively porous-coated stems in revision hip arthroplasty. *Clin Orthop Relat Res*. 1999;369:230-242.
3. Egan KJ, Di Cesare PE. Intraoperative complications of revision hip arthroplasty using a fully porous-coated straight cobalt-chrome femoral stem. *J Arthroplasty*. 1995;10(Suppl):S45-S51.
4. Krishnamurthy AB, MacDonald SJ, Paprosky WG. 5- to 13-year follow-up study on cementless femoral components in revision surgery. *J Arthroplasty*. 1997;12(8):839-847.
5. Chappell JD, Lachiewicz PF. Fracture of the femur in revision hip arthroplasty with a fully porous-coated component. *J Arthroplasty*. 2005;20(2):234-238.
6. Haddad FS, Duncan CP, Berry DJ, Lewallen DG, Gross AE, Chandler HP. Periprosthetic femoral fractures around well-fixed implants: use of cortical onlay allografts with or without a plate. *J Bone Joint Surg Am*. 2002; 84-A(6):945-950.
7. Berry DJ. Treatment of Vancouver B3 periprosthetic femur fractures with a fluted tapered stem. *Clin Orthop Relat Res*. 2003;417:224-231.

SECTION VII

POSTOPERATIVE QUESTIONS

WHEN AND HOW DO I PERFORM AN EXTENDED TROCHANTERIC OSTEOTOMY?

Michael Archibeck, MD

The need for an extended trochanteric osteotomy (ETO) should be anticipated preoperatively. The ETO is helpful in the following instances:

* Primary total hip arthroplasty[1]:
  - Retained intramedullary hardware requiring direct access to remove
  - Mild proximal femoral deformity (ie, varus bow)
* Revision total hip arthroplasty[2,3]
  - Removal of well-fixed cemented or cementless femoral components[4]
  - Femoral revision with difficult cement removal
  - Proximal femoral varus remodeling with a loose femoral component
  - Need for enhanced acetabular exposure
  - Periprosthetic fracture requiring femoral revision
  - Need for more direct visualization of the femoral diaphysis
    - ❖ Generally advantageous with implantation of tapered, fluted revision femoral component

Relative contraindications for the osteotomy include the following:

* Anticipated need for cemented femoral revision
* Impaction grafting

I use the preoperative radiographs to plan the length of the osteotomy. The length of the ETO is a compromise between exposure and preservation of adequate cortical bone distally for fixation of the revision component (usually 4 to 6 cm of intact isthmic diaphysis needed for scratch fit). The distance from the tip of the greater trochanter to distal extent of the ETO is measured with a magnified ruler on preoperative radiographs and recorded for intraoperative reference. I generally perform an ETO between 10 and 16 cm in length depending on the clinical scenario. Most often the osteotomy extends just proximal to the tip of the stem that needs to be removed. If a well-fixed fully porous stem is to be removed, the ETO needs to be performed to the level of the cylindrical portion of the stem in anticipation of stem transection and trephine use.[5]

While the ETO can be performed in association with anterior or direct lateral approaches, I generally use a posterior approach. The posterior soft tissue attachments of the short external rotators and capsule can be left intact but are generally released for improved exposure. The technique for performing the ETO depends on my ability to remove the femoral component easily (as in the case of a polished cemented component or loose component). The ETO is typically performed after dislocation of the hip but can be performed prior to dislocation if a difficult dislocation is anticipated. The fascia of the vastus lateralis is then incised, leaving a 1-cm cuff of fascia posteriorly for closure. The muscle is then divided with particular attention paid to identifying and managing the perforating vessels. I generally release the insertion of the gluteus maximus directly off bone. Once the posterior aspect of the proximal femur is exposed to the desired distance from the tip of the greater trochanter, a Homan retractor is placed anteriorly in a submuscular position at the level of the anticipated transverse portion of the osteotomy. Vastus muscle is elevated in this region to provide adequate exposure but does not need to be elevated more proximally. I generally leave as much of the attachment of the vastus lateralis to the trochanteric fragment intact as possible.

The posterior limb of the ETO is performed with a microsagittal saw from the posterior aspect of the greater trochanter extending distally. Other options include a full-size sagittal saw or a pencil-tipped high-speed bur. If the femoral component has already been removed, the saw can be passed through the medullary canal and the anterior femoral cortex performing the anterior limb of the osteotomy. The ETO should incorporate approximately the lateral third of the femoral diaphyseal circumference. Once the posterior limb has been performed to the planned distance, the distal extent is performed. I generally use a high-speed pencil-tipped burr to perform a rounded and slightly beveled transverse cut. If the anterior limb has not been performed (the femoral component is still in situ), it is initiated distally and proximally using a microsagittal saw. The anterior submuscular portion of the osteotomy can be initiated with a series of drill holes, or, as I like to do, by scoring the anterior cortex with a thin 0.25-inch osteotome from distal to proximal in a submuscular fashion. These techniques will aid in "steering" the controlled anterior fracture to exit at the desired locations proximally and distally. Once complete, I confirm that the corners are complete with a thin 0.25-inch osteotome. Two to 3 large osteotomes are then passed from posterior to anterior and the fragment is gently booked open on its anterior muscular hinge, exposing the underlying component or cement mantle. It is critical, at this point, to release any scar tissue or pseudocapsule anteriorly that typically tethers the proximal portion of the osteotomy. If this is not released, there is a risk of fracture with anterior retraction of the fragment. Once released, broad Bennett-type retractors are placed to retract the ETO fragment anteriorly. I then place a single diaphyseal prophylactic cerclage cable about 1 to 2 cm distal to the ETO to avoid iatrogenic fracture during femoral component preparation and implantation.

Once the work of the revision is complete, the medial aspect of the ETO fragment is contoured with a high-speed burr to accommodate the revision femoral component. The fragment is then reapproximated to the posterior limb of the ETO to avoid anterior displacement of the ETO fragment and anterior impingement with resultant posterior instability. Occasionally anterior capsule or contracted gluteus minimus is released to allow appropriate positioning of the fragment. I secure the fragment using 2 to 4 cerclage cables tightened from distal to proximal. Stability is again tested to confirm no change secondary to impingement. The vastus is closed with a running absorbable suture and posterior soft tissues are reattached to the trochanter if possible. Postoperative management of these patients typically includes touch down weight bearing and no active hip abduction for 6 weeks.

References

1. Della Valle CJ, Berger RA, Rosenberg AG, Jacobs JJ, Sheinkop MB, Paprosky WG. Extended trochanteric osteotomy in complex primary total hip arthroplasty: a brief note. *J Bone Joint Surg Am.* 2003;85-A(12):2385-2390.
2. Younger TI, Bradford MS, Magnus RE, Paprosky WG. Extended proximal femoral osteotomy: a new technique for femoral revision arthroplasty. *J Arthroplasty.* 1995;10(3):329-338.
3. Chen WM, McAuley JP, Engh CA Jr, Hopper RH Jr, Engh CA. Extended slide trochanteric osteotomy for revision total hip arthroplasty. *J Bone Joint Surg Am.* 2000;82(9):1215-1219.
4. Paprosky WG, Weeden SH, Bowling JW Jr. Component removal in revision total hip arthroplasty. *Clin Orthop.* 2001;(393):181-193.
5. Younger TI, Bradford MS, Paprosky WG. Removal of a well-fixed cementless femoral component with an extended proximal femoral osteotomy. *Contemp Orthop.* 1995;30(5):375-380.

I Have a Patient Who Is Complaining of a Leg Length Inequality Following Surgery. What Should I Tell Her?

Charles R. Clark, MD

The best way to approach this question is to anticipate it. Indeed, leg length inequality is a major problem following total hip arthroplasty and it is associated with multiple problems, including nerve palsy, low back pain, and gait abnormalities. Further, it may have medical/legal repercussions. There are basically 3 facets to managing leg length inequality.[1] These include preoperative assessment, intraoperative measures, and postoperative measures.

Leg length issues are a notable concern as evidenced by the fact that the Joint Commission on Accreditation of Health Care Organizations (JCAHO) has defined this as a major event.[2] Edwards et al have shown that patients who have developed a peroneal nerve injury had an average lengthening of 2.7 cm and those who have had a sciatic nerve palsy had an average lengthening of 4.4 cm.[3] Smith[4] concluded that nerve lengthening of as much as 15% to 20% of the resting length of the nerve is safe; however, most agree that there is no truly "safe degree" of leg lengthening.[4] Gurney et al have shown that a leg length change of 2 to 3 cm is the threshold with regard to the effects on most physiologic parameters.[5]

Preoperative assessment starts with asking the patient his or her perception of his or her baseline leg length followed by a measurement of the leg lengths and using blocks as needed to level the pelvis while the patient is standing. Baseline leg lengths are also established on a preoperative radiograph. Typically, patients have an external rotation contracture with osteoarthritis, and it is important to have the involved extremity internally rotated as much as possible to get a more representative view. This is not only helpful for leg lengths but also preoperative templating, which is also an element affecting length. The use of templates is key to assessing not only the size of the implants, but identifying landmarks for bony cuts and placement of both components. Perhaps the most important element of the preoperative management is to educate the patient on the potential trade-offs regarding leg length. Some lengthening may be indicated for a particularly unstable hip. However, it is very helpful to have the patient understand this beforehand. Informed consent should include a discussion of the fact that no intraoperative assessment of leg length is totally accurate.

Intraoperative measures include careful positioning of the patients and identification of bony landmarks prior to making the incision. Intraoperative radiographs and/or fluoroscopy are very helpful in the assessment of limb length. Various landmarks such as determining the relation of the hip femoral head center to the greater trochanter are useful in assessing length changes between baseline and trial/permanent implants. Some have found helpful the use of a marker placed in the pelvis, typically the ilium, and measuring the length from it to some portion on the greater trochanter. This can easily be accomplished with a threaded Steinman pin, which is placed in the ilium, double bent and a mark made on the greater trochanter. It is very important when using a technique that the extremity be placed in the same relative position particularly with respect to abduction when the measure is made. Further, some believe that the so-called schuck test provides some sense of joint stability. A key component of intraoperative evaluation is a stable pelvic reference combined with accurate leg position for measurement.

Postoperatively, it is not unusual for the patient to express a concern that his or her leg is longer. Having the patient anticipate this preoperatively is helpful. Typically, a leg is shortened because of joint space loss and the patient often perceives an increase from his or her baseline. Clinical assessment is key and blocks can be used to assess the limb length as can radiographic assessment. One should not be too quick to proceed with treatment. The best early intervention is patient education. Further, it is helpful for the surgeon to communicate his or her attitude and positive expectation to the physical therapist so that the therapist, surgeon, and patient are all on the same page so to speak. Ranawat and Rodriguez[6] described 14 patients who had a functional leg length inequality postoperatively at 1 month but all had improved by 6 months. Indeed, the use of an early shoe lift may actually forestall the relative relaxing of a pelvic tilt.

Surgery may be a consideration for intractable cases; however, shortening may be associated with a risk of instability. A modification of the femoral head, a change in the femoral component, or a distal femoral osteotomy (which has the advantage of preserving stability) may all be considerations.

Conclusion

This is an important problem that the surgeon should anticipate. Perhaps the major component of management is patient education from the very beginning. Further, it is important that the surgeon does not guarantee equal limb lengths postoperatively; rather, the surgeon should be realistic regarding the possibilities as well as the trade-offs involved, including the need to achieve intraoperative stability. Patient education regarding these issues from the onset is the key to successful management of leg length following total hip arthroplasty.

References

1. Clark CR, Huddleston HD, Schoch EP, Thomas BJ. Leg length discrepancy after total hip arthroplasty. *J Am Acad Orthop Surg.* 2006;14:38-45.
2. Joint Commission on Accreditation of Healthcare Organizations: Ambulatory Care Sentinel Events Statistics—June 24, 2003. Available at: www.jcaho.org. Accessed November 15, 2005.
3. Edwards BN, Tulles HS, Noble PC. Contributory factors and etiology of sciatic nerve palsy in total hip arthroplasty. *Clin Orthop.* 1987;218:136-141.
4. Smith JW. Factors influencing nerve repair II: collateral circulation of peripheral nerves. *Arch Surg.* 1996;93:433.
5. Gurney B, Mermier C, Robergs R, et al. Effects of limb length discrepancy on gait economy and lower extremity muscle activity in older adults. *J Bone Joint Surg Am.* 2001;83:907-915.
6. Ranawat CS, Rodriguez JA. Functional leg length inequality following total hip arthroplasty. *J Arthroplasty.* 1997;12:359-364.

I HAVE A PATIENT WHO IS 2 WEEKS POSTOPERATIVE FROM A PRIMARY TOTAL HIP ARTHROPLASTY AND THE WOUND IS DRAINING. WHAT SHOULD I DO?

Craig J. Della Valle, MD

Some wound drainage is to be expected following total hip arthroplasty (THA). In a study of wound drainage following 1211 primary THAs,[1] the authors found that at 5 days postoperatively, approximately 20% of wounds still had some drainage. Prolonged wound drainage was associated with morbid obesity (body mass index of >40), increased drain output, and the use of low-molecular-weight heparin for thromboembolic prophylaxis. Further, prolonged wound drainage was associated with a statistically significant incidence of deep wound infection and that each day of wound drainage increased the risk of wound infection by over 40%, highlighting the importance of closely monitoring patients in whom the wound drains for more than 5 days.

When presented with the wound that is draining in the early postoperative period, my first concern is determining if there is a deep periprosthetic infection. The use of oral or parenteral antibiotics is discouraged until a definitive diagnosis is made as the indiscriminate use of antibiotics may cloud the clinical picture. Further, skin swabs of a draining wound provide little useful information and should likewise be discouraged.

The diagnosis can be made clinically in some cases. Patients who present with systemic symptoms (such as fever), a wound that is draining purulent fluid with associated erythema (Figure 38-1), and an increasing pain pattern have a deep infection and are brought urgently to the operating room. Similarly, the majority of patients who have scant drainage will oftentimes respond to discontinuing their anticoagulation, local painting of the wound with povidine-iodine, and frequent dressing changes; these patients are, however, carefully instructed to return to the office immediately if their wound drainage changes in quantity or character, if they experience additional pain, or if they develop a fever. Unfortunately, the clinical picture is oftentimes not so clear and in these cases, the

Figure 38-1. Infected hip wound. (Courtesy of J. Parvizi, MD.)

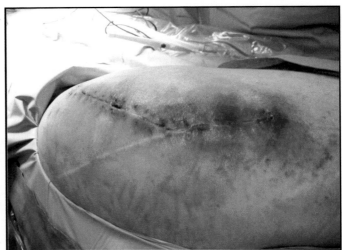

best test available in my experience is an aspiration of the hip done with fluoroscopic guidance.

To perform an aspiration, bring the patient to the fluoroscopy suite and carefully prep an area of the skin remote from the incision and any associated erythema (if present). The aspiration is performed without the use of local anesthesia (as this can act as a bacteriostatic agent) using an 18-gauge spinal needle. The needle is guided into the joint using fluoroscopy, aiming for the prosthetic femoral head. If fluid is obtained, it is sent for a cell count with differential and a full set of cultures (aerobic, anaerobic, fungal, and for acid-fast bacilli). At this point antibiotics can be administered as cultures have been obtained.

In my experience, the cell count and differential are very useful for determining if a deep infection is present. Although limited data are available on the use of synovial fluid white blood cell (WBC) counts in the early postoperative period, prior work from our group[2] has shown that a cell count of greater than 10,000 WBC/mL is consistent with a deep infection while counts of less than 3000 are not and I have used these guidelines in my own clinical practice. Similarly, the differential can be helpful with greater than 90% polymorphonuclear cells consistent with infection although a differential as low as 60% has been associated with infection in some series.[3] If the synovial fluid WBC count is in-between these 2 numbers (3000 and 10,000), I will admit the patient and place him or her on intravenous vancomycin until the results of the cultures are known.[4]

Unfortunately, there will be cases where no fluid can be obtained at the time of aspiration. In these cases, if the drainage is copious, I will bring the patient back to the operating room for a wound exploration as in my mind this either represents an infection, a large hematoma, or a rent in the deep fascia that is allowing joint fluid to escape from the wound; all of these are indications for reoperation. Further, the surgeon should be strongly cautioned against performing a superficial irrigation and debridement if the deep fascia appears intact once the subcutaneous tissues have been opened. If infection is present, it will almost surely connect with the deeper tissues, and if infection is not present, there is little additional risk in reopening the deeper parts of the wound.

The final group of patients is those in whom no fluid can be aspirated from the joint and there is enough drainage to be concerned but not enough to clearly indicate the patient for surgery. In these unusual cases, I will admit the patient to the hospital to monitor him or her closely for systemic symptoms (fever checks every 2 to 4 hours) and to monitor the progress of the wound. Within a day or two, the appropriate course of action is usually clear.

If a deep infection is confirmed, the patient is immediately brought to the operating room. I typically discuss with patients 2 options for operative intervention: irrigation and debridement with an exchange of the modular femoral head and liner or primary removal of the components as the first step in a two-stage exchange. I counsel patients that an irrigation and debridement within the first several weeks following surgery should result in an infection eradication rate of approximately 50% while proceeding directly to a two-stage exchange protocol is associated with eradication of infection in greater than 90% of patients. I am more likely to recommend primary removal of components if the patient is immunocompromised, has other indwelling prosthesis, or if cementless components were used for the index procedure as there is little morbidity associated with their removal (when compared to a cemented femoral stem) and their outcomes (in terms of infection eradication) appear to be worse.[5,6]

References

1. Patel VP, Walsh M, Sehgal B, Preston C, DeWal H, Di Cesare PE. Factors associated with prolonged wound drainage after primary total hip and knee arthroplasty. *J Bone Joint Surg Am.* 2007;89:33-38.
2. Schnisky M, Della Valle C, Sporer S, Paprosky W. Perioperative testing for sepsis in revision total hip arthroplasty. *J Bone Joint Surg Am.* In press.
3. Mason JB, Fehring TK, Odum SM, Griffin WL, Nussman DS. The value of white blood cell counts before revision total knee arthroplasty. *J Arthroplasty.* 2003;18:1038-1043.
4. Fulkerson E, Della Valle CJ, Wise B, Walsh M, Preston C, Di Cesare PE. Antibiotic susceptibility of bacteria infecting total joint arthroplasty sites. *J Bone Joint Surg Am.* 2006;88:1231-1237.
5. Tsukayama DT, Estrada R, Gustilo RB. Infection after total hip arthroplasty: a study of the treatment of one hundred and six infection. *J Bone Joint Surg Am.* 1996;78:512-522.
6. Crockarell JR, Hanssen AD, Osmon DR, Morrey BF. Treatment of infection with debridement and retention of the components following hip arthroplasty. *J Bone Joint Surg Am.* 1998;80:1306-1312.

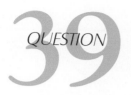

MY PATIENT HAS A FOOT-DROP AFTER SURGERY. WHAT SHOULD I DO?

Marc M. DeHart, MD

Foot drop—the inability to dorsiflex the toes and ankle—is the most common clinical presentation of nerve injury after hip arthroplasty and represents failure of the peroneal division of the sciatic nerve. "Flail foot" is a rare devastating complication that results from complete sciatic nerve lesion with loss of both dorsiflexion and plantarflexion. Sensory loss may involve the entire foot and can lead to reflex sympathetic dystrophy-like changes, pressure sores, infections, and possibly amputations.

The etiology of nerve injury is multifactorial. When measured by electromyography (EMG), 70% of patients have subclinical sciatic nerve damage after total hip arthroplasty (THA). Over 50% of palsy patients have a pre-existing peripheral neuropathy.[1] Patient populations at increased risk include patients with revisions, fibrotic ankylosis after joint sepsis, developmental dysplasia, limb lengthening, post-traumatic arthritis, cementless femoral implant fixation, and those with posterior approaches.[2-4] Fortunately, the prevalence of clinically significant sciatic nerve palsy after hip arthroplasty is only about 0.1% to 0.2%.[2] This rarity provides few evidence-based treatment recommendations. Timely diagnosis and early discussion of possible etiologies and outcomes increases trust in the physician, enhances patient satisfaction, and creates a more positive emotional response in the patient. It also may help minimize potential litigation. Describing the difference between loss of nerve function versus loss of nerve continuity provides a framework for understanding all possible outcomes.[5]

Some recovery of motor function in the first week or 2 after surgery indicates normal or near normal function is likely in longer term follow-up. Complete motor palsy, or complete motor and sensor palsy, indicates a poor prognosis. The largest series of complete nerve palsies noted approximately one-third recovered fully, one-third had partial recovery, and one third had no recovery. Maximal recovery averaged 1 to 2 years.[2] The worst prognosis is found in palsy patients with dysesthesias that develop into complex regional

Figure 39-1.
Supportive care protocol to address clinical problems related to sciatic nerve palsy after total hip arthroplasty.

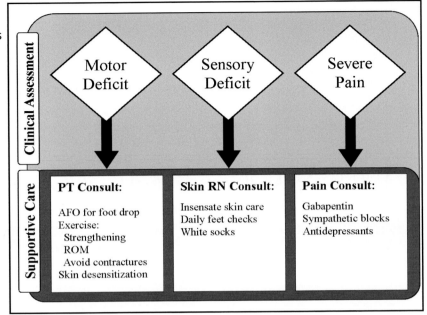

pain syndrome (CRPS). Because most palsy patients enjoy partial or complete recovery, the surgeon should remain hopeful for the patient and the family. The physician should create a specific, proactive rehabilitation plan of care and recruit support of the patient (Figure 39-1).

When foot drop is encountered after THA, avoiding positions of hip flexion with knee extension may help reduce tension on the nerve. Perform a thorough exam and identify the extent of motor and sensory involvement as well as any skin hypersensitivity. Carefully review postoperative radiographs. Continue postoperative rehabilitation as normally as possible. Reviewing the many potential sources of palsy may help guide specific treatment (Table 39-1); however, the etiology is unknown in more than half of cases. When no cause is identified, supportive care of specific deficits is warranted. Motor deficits causing foot drop are best managed with an ankle-foot orthoses (AFO) to allow clearance during the swing phase of gait and to prevent late equinus deformity. Physical therapy is helpful to instruct patients on a home program of ankle dorsiflexor strengthening, plantarflexor stretching to prevent joint contractures, and skin desensitization in cases of causalgia. Sensory deficits demand diligence on the part of the patient to prevent heel ulcers and inadvertent foot trauma. Consultation with a skin care nurse as in patients with diabetic neuropathy may be worthwhile. Patients with dysesthesias and causalgic pain may benefit from pain management consultation and are often helped with gabapentin, antidepressants, and sympathetic nerve blocks.

Certain situations may encourage more immediate management. In the rare case where an obvious mechanical source of compression is identified, it should be removed. Postoperative radiographs can show unexpected posteriorly protruded cement, bony fragments, or proud screws, and exploration may be considered. If postoperative radiographs document excessive lengthening, consider shortening procedures.

Table 39-1
Etiology of Nerve Palsy in Total Hip Arthroplasty

Direct Laceration

- Scalpel/electrocautery
- Retractors
- Wires
- Reamers
- Bone fragments
- Acetabular screws
- Cement protrusion

Direct Compression/Constriction/ Tension

- Retractors
- Subfascial hematoma
- Gluteus maximus insertion
- Piriformis entrapment/retraction
- Dislocation
- Sutures/wires/cables
- Excessive lengthening

Indirect "Double Crush"

- Lumbar stenosis
- Peroneal compression at fibular head
- Pre-existing neuropathy
  - Diabetic
  - Ethanol/alcohol related
  - Hypothyroid
  - Rheumatoid arthritis, systemic lupus erythematosus
  - Vascular neuropathy (nonsystemic vasculitic neuropathy)
    - HIV, hepatitis C, cytomegalovirus
  - Renal disease
  - Liver disease
  - Vitamin deficiency (B_{12})
  - Toxic: styrene, polyvinyl chloride
  - Paraneoplastic

A delayed onset of progressive neurologic symptoms after a normal postoperative check should alert the physician to consider correction of coagulation status and evacuation of a subfascial hematoma. Decreasing neurologic function and unexpected or increasing leg pain with significant buttock or thigh swelling suggest a hematoma in the region of the sciatic nerve. Cases recognized early, and promptly evacuated, show earlier and more complete recovery.[6]

Fortunately, serial examinations over time frequently show some recovery of nerve function. Electromyograms and nerve conduction velocity measurements 6 to 8 weeks after diagnosis provide a more objective measure of the level of injury, the degree of injury, and evidence of recovery of function. In patients whose palsy has not cleared, this also provides an opportunity to document and reinforce compliance with physical therapy, skin nurse, and pain management recommendations. Patients who had symptoms of stenosis prior to arthroplasty and have no recovery of their foot drop by 3 months may benefit from correcting coexisting spinal stenosis.[7] If EMG shows no signs of nerve regeneration by 3 months, consider referral for late surgical exploration. Neurolysis, direct suture repair, and cable grafting techniques may have limited success if performed within 7 months after injury.[8] Since maximal recovery of nerve palsy may take years, the late definitive reconstructive salvage procedures of tendon transfers ("bridle transfer") or ankle fusions should be deferred at least 18 months.

Table 39-2
Pearls to Prevent Palsies

When using posterior retractors:
- Place retractors carefully on bone
- Replace posterior retractors carefully
- Avoid positions of hip flexion and knee extension

Consider sciatic nerve identification, neurolysis, and protection with:
- Revision cases
- Postinfectious arthritis
- Complex cases
- Dissection posterior to acetabulum

When planning lengthening:
- Palpate sciatic nerve to assess tension
- Consider releasing gluteus maximus insertion on femur

When cerclaging femurs:
- Place wires/cables around femur from posterolateral to anterior-medial
- Internally rotate hip to better see posterior femur

In cementless femoral fixation provide counterforce against knee to support femur and avoid repetitive soft tissue traction with stem impaction forces.

Consider anterior/anterolateral approaches.

Prevention

As with all complications, prevention is preferable. Careful attention to detail, gentle handling of soft tissues, awareness of the anatomy, and experience are rewarded with fewer complications (Table 39-2).

References

1. Dellon AL. Postarthroplasty "palsy" and systemic neuropathy: a peripheral-nerve management algorithm. *Ann Plast Surg.* 2005;55(6):638-642.
2. Farrell CM, Springer BD, Haidukewych GJ, Morrey BF. Motor nerve palsy following primary total hip arthroplasty. *J Bone Joint Surg.* 2005;87(12):2619-2625.
3. Pekkarinen J, Alho A, Puusa A, Paavilainen T. Recovery of sciatic nerve injuries in association with total hip arthroplasty in 27 patients. *J Arthroplasty.* 1999;14(3):305-311.
4. Schmalzried TP, Amstutz HC, Dorey FJ. Nerve palsy associated with total hip replacement: risk factors and prognosis. *J Bone Joint Surg Am.* 1991;73(7):1074-1080.
5. DeHart MM, Riley LH Jr. Nerve injuries in total hip arthroplasty. *J Am Acad Orthop Surg.* 1999;7:101-111.
6. Butt AJ, McCarthy T, Kelly IP, Glynn T, McCoy G. Sciatic nerve palsy secondary to postoperative haematoma in primary total hip replacement. *J Bone Joint Surg.* 2005;87-B(11):1465-1467.

7. Pritchett JW. Lumbar decompression to treat foot drop after hip arthroplasty. *Clin Orthop Relat Res.* 1994;303: 173-177.

8. Kim DH, Murovic JA, Tiel R, Kline DG. Management and outcomes in 353 surgically treated sciatic nerve lesions. *J Neurosurg.* 2004;101(1):8-17.

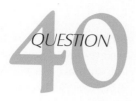
HOW DO YOU MANAGE THE PATIENT WITH AN UNEXPECTEDLY POSITIVE CULTURE AT THE TIME OF A REVISION TOTAL HIP ARTHROPLASTY?

Scott M. Sporer, MD

Is the hip infected or not? This is the question that ultimately is asked once a culture becomes positive following revision hip surgery. Unfortunately, there is no gold standard to define infection. Historically, a positive culture on solid medium has been considered a deep infection, but there are instances of false positives as well as false negatives using this criterion. The true prevalence of false-positive cultures following total joint arthroplasty is extremely variable and has been reported anywhere between 3% and 52%. Most surgeons classify prosthetic joint infections based upon the time of their identification following the index surgical procedure. Type I infections represent a negative preoperative evaluation with an associated positive intraoperative culture. The difficulty again becomes determining what is the definitive test in identifying infection and subsequently determining what represents a true Type I infection versus a false positive. While consultation with an infectious disease specialist is advised when an intraoperative culture is positive, the orthopedic surgeon who performed the hip revision frequently is more knowledgeable of the literature surrounding prosthetic infections.

To begin, the clinical scenario surrounding the hip revision must be considered when deciding the appropriate treatment of a positive intraoperative culture. A thorough history should have been performed prior to the surgical procedure to determine patients who are at an elevated risk for infection. This includes patients with early prosthetic loosening, difficulty with wound healing, or any systemic disease that would cause the patient to be immunocompromised (diabetes, HIV, transplant, medication, etc). Additionally, any preoperative laboratory tests, including a complete blood count (CBC), erythrocyte sedimentation rate (ESR), and/or C-reactive protein (CRP), should be reviewed. While the CBC is frequently normal in patients with an occult hip infection, it is extremely rare that the preoperative ESR and CRP would remain normal. Laboratory tests along with soft tissue samples obtained at the time of revision should also be examined. The synovial cell count is generally elevated in the setting of occult infection with an associated differential showing a predominance of polymorphonucleocytes (PMNs). Additionally, the results of an intraoperative frozen section can be beneficial while the results of intraoperative Gram stains provide little help in making an accurate diagnosis of prosthetic joint infection. Finally, the details surrounding the positive culture must be known. Was the culture positive only in the broth? Was only one culture taken at the time of surgery? How long after the surgery did the result become positive? One colony of growth in the broth only rarely represents true infection and most surgeons would recommend no further treatment.

Currently in my practice, a patient who is at high risk for infection is scheduled for a preoperative hip aspiration. Routine hip aspiration for all patients is not advised especially in the setting of a normal preoperative ESR and CRP. Limiting the preoperative aspiration to high-risk patients will minimize the chance of a false positive by raising the "pretest probability." It is advised that all patients should be off all antibiotics for a minimum of 2 weeks prior to hip aspiration. At the time of surgery, synovial fluid should be sent for a cell count with differential, and tissue surrounding the joint should be sent for frozen section. A synovial cell count greater than 3000 with a differential showing >90% PMN is highly suspicious for infection. Cell counts greater than 10,000 have a high specificity for infection even in patients with a history of autoimmune disease. A frozen section showing an average of greater than 10 PMNs per high power field in the 3 most cellular fields is highly suspicious of infection. Multiple frozen sections should be sent especially if the preoperative ESR, CRP, or intraoperative cell count is elevated. I recommend obtaining a minimum of 3 complete sets of cultures at the time of surgery. Obtaining multiple specimens cannot only help identify a true infection but can also minimize the chances of a false positive. When 3 specimens are obtained, a culture is considered positive when at least 2 of the specimens demonstrate growth on a solid medium. It is advised the culture swabs be opened immediately prior to obtaining the sample rather than having them opened during the initial surgical "set-up."

The recommended treatment of a positive intraoperative culture is heavily dependent upon prior tests. Prolonged antibiotics are not advised if all other laboratory indices are normal (ESR, CRP, cell count, frozen) and only one culture is obtained and shown to be abnormal. In contrast, if all laboratory indices are normal but greater than half of the intraoperative cultures are positive, I advise a 6-week course of antibiotics. Similarly, I advise a 6-week course of antibiotics in patients with a positive culture (any number) and either a cell count >3000, %PMNs >90%, or >10 PMN per high power field. I do not advise acute component resection for a positive culture unless the patient is exhibiting clinical signs of infection in the immediate postoperative period.

Bibliography

Barrack RL, Aggarwal A, Burnett S, et al. The fate of the unexpected positive intraoperative cultures after revision knee arthroplasty. *J Arthroplasty.* 2007;22(6 Supp 2):94-99.

Bauer TW, Parvizi J, Kobayashi N, et al. Diagnosis of periprosthetic infection. *J Bone Joint Surg Am.* 2006;88: 869.

SECTION VIII

FAILED
GENERAL QUESTIONS

I Performed a Hip Revision Using a 20-mm Extensively Coated Stem. At Her 5-Year Follow-Up Appointment She Is Asymptomatic But I See Severe Proximal Bone Loss. Do I Need to Do Anything?

Kevin B. Fricka, MD

The simple answer to this question is no, the surgeon does not need to do anything. The patient is asymptomatic with a well-ingrown femoral stem. As my standard, routine annual follow-up to assess for signs of polyethylene wear, osteolysis, or loosening is all that I recommend.

However, in order to answer this question, the orthopedic surgeon must be familiar with the concepts of distal fixation and proximal stress shielding. As in this case, the goals with the use of a cementless extensively porous-coated stem for femoral revision are initial diaphyseal stability and subsequent osseointegration for long-term stability. With the insertion of a stemmed prosthesis into the femur, adaptive bone remodeling begins to take place and can lead to varying degrees of bone loss.[1] This bone remodeling is a ubiquitous phenomenon that occurs with all types of cemented and noncemented femoral stems. When using an extensively porous-coated cementless stem, distal fixation of the prosthesis in the diaphysis is achieved. With distal fixation and osseointegration, the mechanical stress level within the proximal bone is decreased. Thus resorption occurs as governed by the principles of Wolff's law; bone remodeling occurs in response to the degree of mechanical stress placed upon it. This stress-mediated bone resorption that is visible radiographically is defined as stress shielding.[1]

Stress shielding occurs with all types of hip arthroplasty implants to varying degrees in different patients. Risk factors that are associated with stress shielding include bone quality, stem size, extent of porous coating, gender, and age. Bone quality is best assessed by measuring the cortical index, a ratio of the periosteal femoral diameter to the endosteal femoral diameter measured at the diaphysis. Stress shielding is more prevalent in patients with a lower cortical index and thus patients are graded with a poorer bone quality. Large diameter stem size with increasing stiffness is also correlated with stress shielding; however, this is not a linear relationship. The bending rigidity of the cylindrical portion of the implant increases directly with the fourth power of its diameter, so for every 1 mm increase in stem diameter there is a fourth power increase in stiffness.[2] Thus the worst situation from a stress-shielding perspective would be a large stem diameter placed into a femur with thin cortices. The extent of porous coating has an influence on the degree of stress shielding as well. Extensively porous-coated stems tend to funnel more load distally and stress relieve more bone proximally.[2] Age and female gender are secondary risk factors in that the tendency is for older, female patients to present with larger intramedullary canals and thinner cortices (lower cortical index), thus leading to the use of larger diameter extensively porous-coated implants and an increase in the degree of stress shielding.

Clinical problems directly attributable to proximal femoral stress-related bone resorption have not been reported with any significant frequency in the literature. Dr. William Harris in his paper about stress shielding and longevity expressed some concerns when faced with proximal femoral bone loss in a well-functioning total hip arthroplasty.[3] He felt that stress shielding created a high stress area at the end of the porous coating where dense cortical bone ingrowth occurs. This was believed to expose the implant to cantilever forces that may predispose to stem fracture, thigh pain, or late femoral component loosening. Secondly, he felt that proximal bone loss could increase the patient's risk of pathologic periprosthetic fractures and complicate revision surgery when attempting to remove well-fixed components from osteoporotic bone. The third consideration was the concept that stress-shielded bone may be more susceptible to particle-induced osteolysis.

These concerns were addressed in a long-term follow-up paper done at this institution (Anderson Orthopedic Clinic) that evaluated the clinical outcomes of a group of 48 THAs with radiographically evident stress shielding compared with 160 control THAs.[4] In this study, there were no broken femoral components or late loosening in the stress-shielded group and the incidence of thigh pain was not different between the 2 groups. Stress shielding and bony spot welds are signs of osseointegration and late loosening was not a concern at 14.3 years follow-up. There was no difference in the occurrence of periprosthetic fractures between the groups. The removal of these components in the face of severe stress shielding can pose a challenge and there is a risk of femoral fracture. In this study there were no femoral revisions in the group with stress shielding; however, the removal of extensively coated stems can be accomplished without complication by using good surgical technique, an extended trochanteric osteotomy, a metal cutting burr to cut the stem, and trephines to remove the distal stem. Patients with stress shielding also did not demonstrate a difference in the occurrence of femoral osteolysis and were less likely to undergo reoperation for polyethylene wear and osteolysis. The typical patient with stress shielding is a lighter weight, older female patient who had a large diameter stem

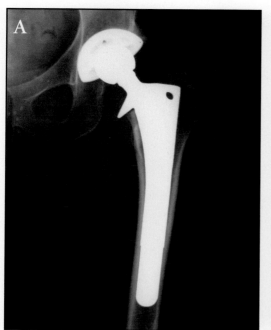
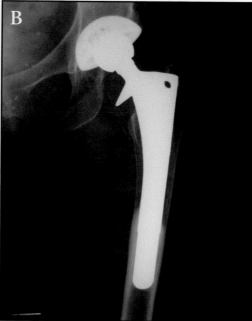

Figure 41-1. (A) Immediate postoperative and (B) 6-year follow-up x-rays demonstrating severe stress shielding in this 74-year-old female s/p total hip arthroplasty. This patient had several risk factors for stress shielding to include age, gender, low cortical index, large stem size (19.5 mm), and an extensively porous-coated implant. At 6-year follow-up, signs of stable osseointegration are demonstrated with distal bony spot welds and calcar resorption. Clinically the patient is doing excellent without limitations.

inserted. Thus this lower demand group was likely protected from significant problems with wear and osteolysis.

My recommendation for this patient is continued routine follow-up with performance of her activities as tolerated. I use this femoral design (extensively porous-coated implants) in the revision setting because it provides predictable long-term fixation with good clinical results and high patient satisfaction (Figure 41-1). Concerns of clinical significance in the presence of stress shielding have not been demonstrated in the literature. Stress shielding is no more than a radiographic finding consistent with a well-ingrown femoral implant. Complications related to wear and osteolysis are a much greater problem than stress shielding of the femur.

References

1. Bobyn JD, Mortimer ES, Glassman AH, et al. Producing and avoiding stress shielding: laboratory and clinical observations of noncemented total hip arthroplasty. *Clin Orthop.* 1992;274:79-96.
2. Engh CA, Bobyn JD. The influence of stem size and extent of porous coating on femoral bone resorption after primary cementless hip arthroplasty. *Clin Orthop.* 1988;231:7-28.
3. Harris WH. Will stress-shielding limit the longevity of cemented femoral components of total hip replacement? *Clin Orthop.* 1992;274:120-123.
4. Engh CA Jr, Young AM, Engh CA Sr, Hopper RH Jr. Clinical consequences of stress shielding after porous-coated total hip arthroplasty. *Clin Orthop.* 2003;417:157-163.

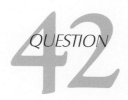

A 74-Year-Old Patient Has Failed Two Attempted Two-Stage Exchanges for Infection and Continues to Have Purulent Drainage From the Wound. When Do You Use Antibiotic Suppression and When Do You Perform a Resection Arthroplasty?

W. Randall Schultz, MD, MS
J. Todd Bagwell, MD

This patient has clearly demonstrated failure to eradicate the infection and sterilize the hip joint thus leading to repetitive failures of reimplantation due to infection. We would first make certain that the prior two-stage exchange procedures were performed adequately both in terms of surgical and medical treatment. The surgical debridement should adequately remove all hardware, cement, and devitalized bone or bone graft material. Interim antibiotic spacers have also been shown to increase the efficacy of antibiotic treatment by providing local antibiotic concentrations that exceed that provided by parenteral therapy.[1] It is also wise to review the culture data. Specifically, one should make sure adequate cultures have been performed and that suitable antimicrobials were utilized in treatment. The medical treatment should include at a minimum 4 weeks of parenteral antibiotic therapy particularly when more virulent organisms are involved (Table 42-1).[2]

If these conditions have been met, then it is unlikely that repeat two-stage exchange will be effective in eradicating the infection. At that point, one would need to consider

Table 42-1
Virulence of Casual Microorganisms

Less Virulent

- *Staphylococcus epidermidis* (methicillin-susceptible)
- *Staphylococcus aureus* (methicillin-susceptible)
- Anaerobic Gram-positive cocci
- Streptococci (other than enterococci)
- *P. acnes*

More Virulent

- Gram-negative bacilli (particularly *Pseudomonas*)
- *Staphylococcus epidermidis* (methicillin-susceptible)
- *Staphylococcus aureus* (methicillin-sensitive)
- Group D streptococci (enterococci)
  - *Candida sp.*
  - Mycobacteria
  - Fungi

Adapted from Clegg J. The results of the pseudoarthrosis after removal of an infected total hip prosthesis. *J Bone Joint Surg Br.* 1977;59(3):298.

long-term antibiotic suppression or resection arthroplasty (Girdlestone procedure). We would base our treatment decision upon several factors:

* The activity level of the patient

* Implant fixation

* The medical condition of the patient

* The virulence of the organism involved

* Ability of the patient to tolerate long-term antibiotic therapy

If the patient is nonambulatory or unlikely to become ambulatory, then we would strongly consider resection arthroplasty particularly if there is significant bone loss or painful loosening. It is well documented that Girdlestone arthroplasty compromises functional outcome in terms of energy expenditure, ambulatory capacity, and leg length discrepancy, but it can be a definitive means of sterilizing the hip.[3-7] It should be used with caution in the medically compromised patient as frequently the length of surgery and blood loss involved can be significant, with one series reporting an average blood loss of 2400 mL and an average operative time of 188 minutes.[6] If the patient is not medically fit for an extensive surgical procedure, then we would first attempt antibiotic suppression regardless of activity level.

If the patient has a relatively well-fixed implant and functional status allows for at least limited ambulation, then we would consider antibiotic suppression if the infectious agent is of lesser virulence (see Table 42-1), susceptible to oral antibiotic agents, and lacks biofilm production.[8] Consultation with infectious disease specialists would be essential at this stage in providing guidance as to effective antibiotic treatment and the ability of the patient to tolerate long-term antibiotics and their respective adverse effects. The life expectancy of the patient will need to be considered as well as long-term antibiotics can be associated with drug-resistant superinfections, antibiotic-related colitis, and the development of allergic reactions.

If suitable conditions for antibiotic suppression are not available, then we would at that point revert to considering resection arthroplasty as the definitive treatment. If the patient is medically unfit for surgery and oral suppressive agents are not feasible, then one would have to consider intravenous suppression and limited serial debridements until he or she is medically stable enough to tolerate a major surgical procedure.

References

1. Hanssen AD, Rand JA. Evaluation and treatment of infection at the site of a total hip or knee arthroplasty. *Instr Course Lect.* 1999;48:111-122.
2. McDonald DJ, Fitzgerald RH Jr, Ilstrup DM. Two-stage reconstruction of a total hip arthroplasty because of infection. *J Bone Joint Surg Am.* 1989;1(6):828-834.
3. Bourne RB, Hunter GA, Rorabeck CH, Macnab JJ. A six-year follow-up of infected total hip replacements managed by Girdlestone's arthroplasty. *J Bone Joint Surg Br.* 1984;66(3):340-343.
4. Clegg J. The results of the pseudoarthrosis after removal of an infected total hip prosthesis. *J Bone Joint Surg Br.* 1977;59(3):298-301.
5. Haddad FS, Masri BA, Garbuz DS, Duncan CP. The treatment of the infected hip replacement: the complex case. *Clin Orthop Relat Res.* 1999;369:144-156.
6. Petty W, Goldsmith S. Resection arthroplasty following infected total hip arthroplasty. *J Bone Joint Surg Am.* 1980;62(6):889-896.
7. Waters RL, Perry J, Conaty P, Lunsford B, O'Meara P. The energy cost of walking with arthritis of the hip and knee. *Clin Orthop Relat Res.* 1987;214:278-284.
8. Donlan RM. Biofilm formation: a clinically relevant microbiological process. *Clin Infect Dis.* 2001;33(8):1387-1392.

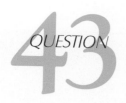

QUESTION

43

I HAVE A PATIENT WITH RECURRENT HIP DISLOCATION AND I THINK THERE IS NOT ENOUGH ANTEVERSION IN THE ACETABULAR COMPONENT. HOW CAN I DETERMINE THE AMOUNT OF FEMORAL AND ACETABULAR ANTEVERSION?

R. Stephen J. Burnett, MD, FRCS(C)
Robert L. Barrack, MD

Dislocation is a frequent early complication of total hip arthroplasty[1] (THA) and is associated with a higher mortality rate compared with THA patients who do not sustain a dislocation.[2] Dislocation is one of the most common causes for revision surgery after loosening and infection.[3] The incidence of dislocation after primary THA within the first 90 days is approximately 3%, while that of revisions is over 2 times higher, and 8%.[4] Most published studies are from high-volume medical centers, yet most hip replacements are done by surgeons who perform a lesser volume of hip arthroplasties. Because of evidence that dislocation rate may be associated with surgeon experience, the incidence of dislocation overall may be higher than is reported from large centers.

The patient who develops recurrent dislocation of a THA presents a challenging problem for the orthopedic surgeon. Patient, surgical, and implant factors have been recognized as contributors to recurrent instability. Multiple etiologies have been recognized to contribute to dislocation in THA, including surgical approach (with the posterolateral approach frequently reported in association with higher dislocation rates than the anterolateral Hardinge approach), abductor deficiency, inadequate offset, multiple prior hip surgeries, impingement (bony, implant, or a combination), infection, polyethylene wear, implant design, and component malposition/malrotation.[5] This chapter will address the

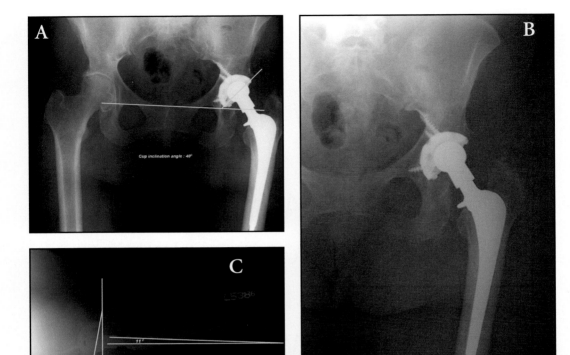

Figure 43-1. (A) AP pelvis x-ray of a left THA. The inclination angle (40 degrees) is calculated by drawing a line joining the 2 teardrops. The inclination of the cup is then drawn, and the inclination angle is created. Note the ellipse representing the acetabular face is wider on the AP pelvis (A) than on the AP hip radiograph (B), thus the acetabulum is retroverted. AP hip x-ray. The ellipse representing the acetabular face should be wider on the AP hip than the AP pelvis, which it is not (retroversion) in this case. (C) Cross-table lateral x-ray (also known as "shoot-through lateral"). The acetabular anteversion is calculated. In this case the acetabular component is retroverted 15 degrees. The femoral component anteversion may be estimated, and on this view measures 11 degrees. This patient had undergone the left THA performed through the antero-lateral approach, which may be associated with less anteversion of the components.

radiographic imaging techniques to address acetabular component position, including anteversion, with the use of plain radiographs and computed tomography (CT) scan.

The approach to this problem begins with a careful history of the hip and the instability, physical examination, and review of prior operative reports and implant records. We find the active side-lying abduction test a reliable indicator and particularly useful clinical test to assess the abductor function in instability cases. Prior radiographs of the hip should be sought and reviewed to determine the direction of dislocation of the hip. A current series of radiographs should be obtained, and we recommend a standing anterior-posterior (AP) pelvis, AP hip, cross table (shoot-through) lateral, and a frog lateral. It is important to establish the acetabular component inclination angle on the AP view (Figure 43-1A), with a "safe zone"[6] described from 30 to 50 degrees of inclination. Ideally, we prefer a cup inclination of 40 to 45 degrees, and with the use of newer cross-linked polyethylenes or hard bearings (metal-metal, ceramic-ceramic), wear and fatigue of the bearing surface are improved at angles of inclination less than 45 degrees and avoiding vertical cup placement. Notably, the fractures that have been reported with cross-linked polyethylene liners are associated with higher inclination angles and recurrent dislocation adjacent to a lipped liner. Computer modeling studies indicate the optimal cup position is 45 to 55 degrees abduction. Angles <55 degrees require anteversion of 10 to 20 degrees of both the stem and cup to minimize the risk of impingement and dislocation.

Once the inclination has been calculated, the acetabular component anteversion is assessed. If the ellipse representing the acetabular face is wider on the AP hip than on the AP pelvis radiograph, the acetabulum is anteverted (Figure 43-1B). We use the cross-table lateral radiograph to assess the acetabular anteversion in all cases, and a CT scan is rarely necessary. There are 3 definitions of acetabular version: true (anatomic) version, planar (radiographic) version, and operative version. Although the planar version can be measured on standard radiographs, the measurement may be inaccurate when applied to metal-backed acetabular components. There have been reports of using the AP radiograph to calculate anteversion with the use of complex trigonometric calculations[6]; however, this is impractical in the clinical setting. The cross-table lateral view is extremely useful and readily distinguishes anteversion from retroversion of the acetabular component (Figure 43-1C). If the angle of the x-ray beam is known and standardized, version measured on the shoot-through lateral of the acetabulum closely approximates planar anteversion.[7] The cross-table lateral view of the hip is obtained with a horizontal x-ray beam aimed at the groin and angled approximately 30 degrees in a cephalad direction. Flexion of the contralateral hip excludes it from the radiograph. The acetabular anteversion angle is drawn between the projected long axis of the acetabular opening and the anteroposterior axis (see Figure 43-1C). This is an approximation only, requiring a vertical patella orientation and is unpublished. In addition, if the leg and foot are oriented with the patella pointing vertically, the femoral component version may be approximated on the same cross-table lateral view (see Figure 43-1C). Important in the consideration of the assessment of anteversion of the femoral and acetabular components is the prior surgical approach used for the surgery. Typically, the anterolateral approach to the hip requires and results in less anteversion of both the femoral and acetabular components, while the posterolateral approach requires more combined anteversion of the components. This is an important consideration when you plan to revise the hip for recurrent dislocation, as the surgical approach and anteversion of the components may be a factor in your decision-making process.

In instances when there is uncertainty about the assessment or technique of anteversion using the cross-table lateral plain radiograph (Figure 43-2), the use of a CT scan[8] may be helpful in determining the anteversion of the acetabular and femoral components. A CT scan is most commonly used in our THA revisions to assess retroacetabular osteolysis. We have on occasion found it more useful to use the CT scan to calculate femoral component anteversion, as the cross-table lateral view is reliable for assessment of acetabular version. Both femoral and acetabular anteversion may be calculated using a CT scan. We have modified the CT technique that has been described for component malrotation in total knee replacement surgery[9] and use a similar protocol for assessment of THA anteversion. We collaborate closely with our musculoskeletal radiologist when a CT of a THA is ordered to assess component version. The technique involves obtaining a CT scan of the

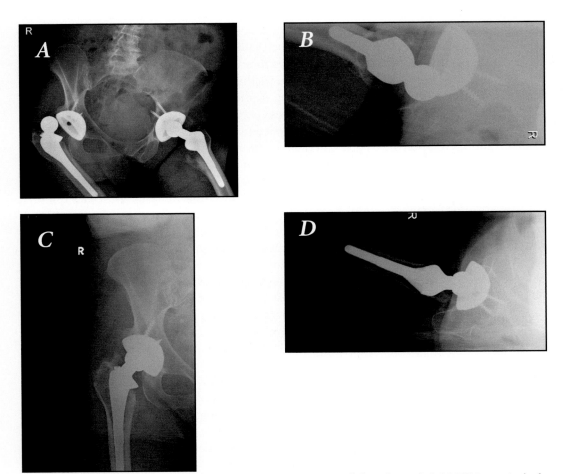

Figure 43-2. AP pelvis x-ray (A) demonstrating recurrent dislocation of right THA, posteriorly (B). AP hip x-ray (C) and cross-table lateral view (D) following closed reduction. The acetabular component appears to be anteverted as seen on the cross-table view, with minimal anteversion of the femoral component.

pelvis and hip, and additional axial cuts at the distal femur in the region of the epicon-dylar axis. Techniques to reduce metal artifact and scatter enhance the CT quality. To calculate the degree of femoral component anteversion, the epicondylar axis (Figure 43-3A) and axis along the neck of the femoral component (Figure 43-3B) are drawn separately in different axial CT cuts, then are superimposed, and the relative anteversion of the femoral neck if the implant in relation to the epicondylar axis provides the femoral component anteversion. Similarly, to assess the degree of acetabular anteversion,[8] the anteroposterior axis of the pelvis is drawn, and the central axis of the acetabular component opening drawn. The acetabular component anteversion may then be calculated by superimposing these 2 axes to create the anteversion angle (Figure 43-3C).

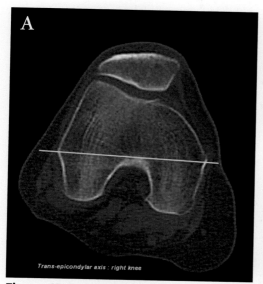
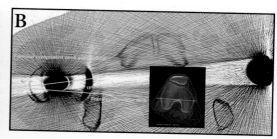
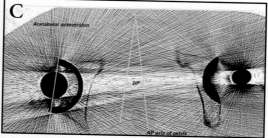

Figure 43-3. CT scan of patient in Figure 43-2 to further assess component version. (A) Calculation of femoral component anteversion. The transepicondylar axis line is drawn first, requiring the CT scan to include cuts in this region of the knee. (B) The CT scan through the neck of the femoral component is used to determine the axis of the femoral anteversion. The epicondylar axis is then transposed to this same image to calculate the femoral component anteversion. (C) The acetabular component anteversion angle is formed by the axis of the acetabular component and the AP axis of the pelvis. The CT scan in this instance confirms the cross-table x-ray findings of an anteverted acetabular component and a minimally anteverted femoral component.

Conclusion

The use of the cross-table radiograph of the hip provides a useful and simple technique to assess acetabular component version, while the AP view determines acetabular inclination. In rare circumstances, the use of CT scan to assess femoral and acetabular anteversion may provide additional information when the plain radiographs are equivocal. The concept of combined component position, in which anteversion and abduction of the acetabular component, along with femoral anteversion, are all combined as critical elements for stability of a THA.

References

1. Paterno SA, Lachiewicz PF, Kelley SS. The influence of patient-related factors and the position of the acetabular component on the rate of dislocation after total hip replacement. *J Bone Joint Surg Am.* 1997;79:1202-1210.
2. Hedlundh U, Fredin H. Patient characteristics in dislocations after primary total hip arthroplasty: 60 patients compared with a control group. *Acta Orthop Scand.* 1995;66:225-228.
3. Eftekhar N. Dislocation and instability. In: Eftekhar NS, ed. *Total Hip Arthroplasty.* St. Louis, MO: Mosby-Year Book; 1993:1505-1553.
4. Mahoned NN, Barrett JA, Katz JN, et al. Rates and outcomes of primary and revision total hip replacement in the United States. *J Bone Joint Surg Am.* 2003;85:27-32.
5. Barrack RL. Dislocation after total hip arthroplasty: implant design and orientation. *J Am Acad Orthop Surg.* 2003;11:89-99.

6. Lewinnek GE, Lewis JL, Tarr R, Compere CL, Zimmerman JR. Dislocations after total hip-replacement arthroplasties. *J Bone Joint Surg Am*. 1978;60:217-220.

7. Yao L, Yao J, Gold RH. Measurement of acetabular version on the axiolateral radiograph. *Clin Orthop Relat Res*. 1995;316:106-111.

8. Mian SW, Truchly G, Pflum FA. Computed tomography measurement of acetabular cup anteversion and retroversion in total hip arthroplasty. *Clin Orthop Relat Res*. 1992;276:206-209.

9. Berger RA, Crossett LS, Jacobs JJ, Rubash HE. Malrotation causing patellofemoral complications after total knee arthroplasty. *Clin Orthop Relat Res*. 1998;356:144-153.

How Do You Evaluate a Patient With a Painful Total Hip Arthroplasty?

Alexander Siegmeth, MD, FRCS
Donald S. Garbuz, MD, FRCSC

Patient outcome after total hip arthroplasty is high, with the vast majority reporting significant improvement in their quality of life and level of function. However, some patients will either not be satisfied postoperatively or present later with new onset of pain and/or reduced level of function. In the majority of these cases, the diagnosis is relatively easy to make with history, clinical examination, blood tests, and radiographs.

Nevertheless, a systematic and structured approach to the patient presenting with a painful total hip arthroplasty is necessary. A successful outcome depends foremost on correct identification of the underlying problem that caused the hip to fail.

Our evaluation begins with the history and physical examination. We take a thorough history that helps us put the problem into a certain category. The pain history is important as the intensity, location, and duration point toward possible etiologies. Unrelenting pain especially during the night combined with a history of prolonged wound healing or drainage makes the diagnosis of infection very likely. We always ask about pain in other areas of the body. Spinal stenosis or discogenic back pain can radiate into the hip and leg.

The physical examination must be comprehensive and covers both hips, knees, and the lumbar spine. We look for antalgic gait, short leg gait, and fixed deformities. Local inspection can reveal scars from previous surgeries, sinuses, and inflammation. Palpation and active and passive movements provide further clues. A neurological and vascular examination is mandatory (sciatic and femoral nerve, nerve root tension signs).

We have now already gained valuable information and this helps us to order the appropriate investigations. Our broad categories are intrinsic causes related to the arthroplasty itself (infection, aseptic loosening, impending periprosthetic fracture, osteolysis, instability, wear debris synovitis) and extrinsic causes (spine disease, tumors, vascular disease, nerve injury, hernias, etc).

All patients must have an anteroposterior radiograph of the pelvis, an anteroposterior and lateral view of the hip, and a lateral radiograph of the femur. Old radiographs often give useful information as some signs are subtle and develop slowly with time.

If cemented implants are in place, we look for definitive signs of loosening such as migration or fracture of the stem or cement mantle or a continuous radiolucent line at the cement-bone interface.[1] If a cementless implant is in place, we look for absence of reactive lines, presence of endosteal spot welds, and absence of a pedestal as signs for osseointegration.[2] Criteria for solid ingrowth of a cementless socket are absence of radiolucent lines, medial stress shielding, presence of superolateral buttress, and radial trabeculae.[3] If we suspect infection, we look for endosteal scalloping, osteolysis, and periosteal new bone formation. Liner wear is also a feature to look out for as this can lead to painful wear debris-induced synovitis or osteolysis with risk of fracture. We use nuclear imaging (Technetium 99) infrequently as it is nonspecific and positive in a variety of conditions such as infection, fracture, and aseptic loosening. Technetium scans remain positive for up to 24 months after surgery. We reserve ultrasound, computed tomography, and magnetic resonance imaging for very specific questions.

The next step is to order basic blood tests. These include complete blood cell count, erythrocyte sedimentation rate (ESR), and C-reactive protein (CRP). CRP and ESR combined are very useful as with a CRP<10 and ESR<30, we can virtually exclude an infection.[4]

Hip aspiration is another useful diagnostic tool. We do not use it in every case of hip pain as it has poor specificity when performed routinely. It has proven to be more sensitive and specific when there is clinical and radiographic evidence of infection or elevation of either CRP or ESR. At the time of aspiration, cultures and a synovial biopsy should be taken and local anesthetic injected when hip and lumbar spine disease coexist.

Conclusion

In the presence of loose implants on radiographs, we rely on CRP and ESR. If they are normal, we proceed to a single-stage revision for aseptic loosening. If they are elevated, we aspirate the hip joint. If that is positive, we do a two-stage revision. If the aspirate is negative and clinically infection is suspicious, we proceed to a single-stage revision with frozen section. If the implants are stable on radiographs, we proceed as above to exclude infection. If that is negative, we try to exclude extrinsic causes and we also consider a bone scan (Technetium 99, Indium).

References

1. O'Neill DA, Harris WH. Failed total hip arthroplasty: assessment by plain radiographs, arthrograms and aspiration of the hip joint. *J Bone Joint Surg Am.* 1984;66:540-546.
2. Engh CA, Massin P, Suthers KE. Roentgenographic assessment of the biologic fixation of porous-surface femoral components. *Clin Orthop Relat Res.* 1990;257:107-128.
3. Moore MS, McAuley JP, Young AM, Engh CA. Radiographic signs of osseointegration in porous coated acetabular components. *Clin Orthop Relat Res.* 2006;444:176-183.
4. Spangehl MJ, Masri BA, O'Connell JX, Duncan CP. Prospective analysis of preoperative and intraoperative investigations for the diagnosis of infection at the sites of 202 revision total hip arthroplasties. *J Bone Joint Surg Am.* 1999;81:672-683.

SECTION IX

FAILED
ACETABULUM QUESTIONS

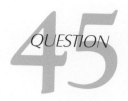
I Have a Patient Who Requires a Polyethylene Liner Revision and Has Minimal Anteversion in His Component. What Surgical Approach Do You Use When Performing an Isolated Polyethylene Liner Exchange?

William V. Arnold, MD, PhD
William J. Hozack, MD

Our favored surgical approach for performing an isolated polyethylene liner exchange is a direct lateral approach. This surgical approach offers a lower postoperative dislocation rate compared with other surgical approaches. It is also a good utilitarian surgical approach for revision surgery generally should the acetabular or the femoral component require revision as determined at the time of surgery. The lower dislocation rate of this approach is important because of the relatively high dislocation rate (up to 25%) reported in the literature for this surgical procedure.[1,2] Our reported dislocation rate with the direct lateral approach is 6% involving 2 of 35 patients at a minimum follow-up of 2 years.[3] Others have also reported good results in terms of postoperative stability with the direct lateral approach.[4] Careful attention to preservation of the soft tissues and closure of the hip joint pseudocapsule may help to minimize the risk of postoperative instability regardless of which surgical approach is chosen.

Beyond the specific surgical approach chosen, there are other important factors to consider for the success of this procedure. Isolated liner exchange should ideally only be done in the setting of a well-fixed, well-positioned acetabular component. Acetabular components that are malpositioned should be considered for component revision, even if there has not been a problem with instability in the past. Other considerations at the time

Figure 45-1. Radiograph of a 77-year-old woman who is 12 years status post right total hip arthroplasty. She presented with a recent onset of recurrent dislocations.

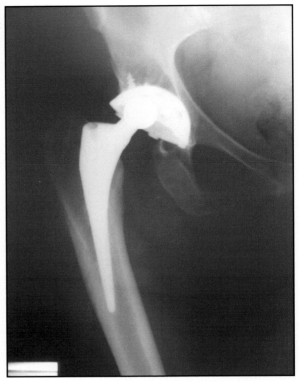

of surgery with regard to retaining the acetabular component include the competence of the liner locking mechanism, the track record of the acetabular component, the availability of a replacement liner, the modularity of the acetabular component, and the quality of the acetabular component. For failed locking mechanisms, cemented acetabular liners are a good option. However, damaged acetabular components, even if well fixed, may not be able to adequately hold a liner, even if it is cemented in place. The decision to remove the acetabular component, however, should not be taken lightly. One may regret this decision, if made for marginal reasons, since removal of a cementless acetabular component may result in significant bone loss and possible fracture. Nonetheless, preoperative planning should always take into account this worst-case scenario with the availability of appropriate materials such as bone allografts and antiprotrusio cages.

Once the decision has been made intraoperatively for an isolated liner exchange (Figure 45-1), any acetabular screws should be removed. Bone defects are then débrided and grafted, although this is not absolutely essential. Other steps must then be taken to help ensure postoperative stability. We do not hesitate to use a larger femoral head for this purpose since larger femoral heads have been shown to improve postoperative stability generally in total hip arthroplasty. With the better cross-linked polyethylene liners now available, we would not hesitate to use a femoral head-acetabular liner combination that has a polyethylene thickness of 6 mm. Elevated rim and offset liners are also an option. Certainly femoral offset as well as head size can also be increased with the femoral head chosen. For these reasons it is imperative to know the identity of the implants from the previous

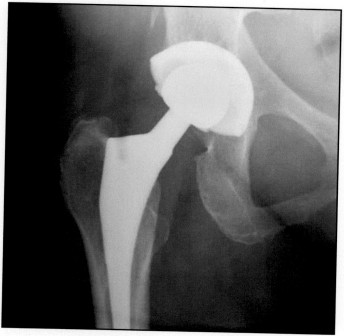

Figure 45-2. Postoperative radiograph following polyethylene liner exchange. Note the removal of previous acetabular screws and the use of a larger femoral head.

surgery preoperatively by obtaining appropriate records. Usually the combination of a larger femoral head with appropriate offset will provide good hip stability as tested intraoperatively (Figure 45-2). Given the high rate of postoperative instability related to this surgical procedure, it is imperative to obtain good stability intraoperatively. Finally, as noted above, the hip pseudocapsule can be preserved with the surgical approach and then closed at the end of the surgery to further promote stability.

Postoperatively, protecting patients with bracing is an option, although we do not routinely do this. It should be noted that with isolated liner exchange, patients will often recover at an accelerated pace and may be less likely to follow hip precautions. It may be necessary to encourage patients to ambulate with assistance for 4 to 6 weeks since they otherwise may not do this on their own.

Conclusion

Our largest concerns with an isolated polyethylene liner exchange involve postoperative stability. The surgical procedure itself is relatively straightforward, although the surgeon must be prepared for the worst-case scenario of removal of the acetabular component and all that this may entail. We try to minimize the problems of postoperative instability with this procedure by using a direct lateral approach and by maximizing the size of the femoral head within the constraints of the acetabular component in place.

References

1. Boucher HR, Lynch C, Young AM, Engh CA Jr, Engh CA Sr. Dislocation after polyethylene liner exchange in total hip arthroplasty. *J Arthroplasty.* 2003;18:654-657.
2. Lachiewicz PF, Soileau ES. Polyethylene liner exchange of the Harris-Galante porous I and II acetabular components without cement: results and complications. *J Arthroplasty.* 2006;21:992-997.
3. Wade FA, Rapuri VR, Parvizi J, Hozack WJ. Isolated acetabular polyethylene exchange through the anterolateral approach. *J Arthroplasty.* 2004;19:498-500.
4. O'Brien JJ, Burnett RS, McCalden RW, MacDonald SJ, Bourne RB, Rorabeck CH. Isolated liner exchange in revision total hip arthroplasty: clinical results using the direct lateral surgical approach. *J Arthroplasty.* 2004;19:414-423.

46

I Have a Patient Who Has Recurrent Hip Instability and the Components Appear Well Fixed and in Appropriate Position. What Should I Do?

Devon D. Goetz, MD

My first step in the evaluation of this particular patient is to obtain extensive information with a medical history, examination, and radiographic evaluation. Specific goals of this process are to determine the direction of hip dislocation, verify that the implants actually are in good position, and ultimately to create a treatment strategy with multiple back-up plans.

Prior to the initial evaluation, we attempt to obtain copies of the patient's implant records, surgical reports, and previous radiographs, including ideally a lateral radiograph when the hip was dislocated. Frequently, these radiographs are not available; therefore, we obtain information regarding the mechanism of dislocation. Usually, posterior dislocations will occur when the hip is flexed (patient sitting), and anterior dislocations will occur when the hip is extended (patient standing). However, this information is unreliable, and the direction of dislocation must be confirmed at the time of surgical exploration. Leg lengths are evaluated by patient impression, standing exam of pelvis obliquity, and radiographs of the pelvis, and I attempt to determine if the patient would be bothered by lengthening of the involved side.

Computed tomography (CT) scans are more accurate in determining implant position than plain radiographs, but we rarely obtain these because the definitive test for implant position is range of motion testing during the intraoperative exam. The anterior-posterior (AP) pelvis and cross-table (shoot-through) lateral is reviewed, and acetabular components near 45 degrees of abduction and 20 degrees of anteversion are considered appropriate (Figure 46-1). In addition to implant fixation status, it is also important to determine the amount of acetabular bone remaining in case a well-fixed acetabular component must be removed.

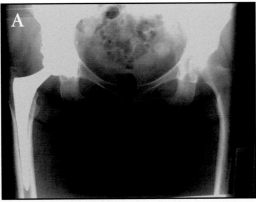

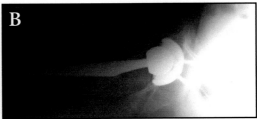

Figure 46-1. Plain radiographs of a primary uncemented total hip replacement. This patient had an anterolateral approach to the hip. In hips that are exposed with an anterior capsular incision, I like to position the acetabular component in approximately 45 degrees of abduction and just under 20 degrees of anteversion. Conversely, in hips that are exposed with a posterior capsular incision, I like to position the acetabular component in at least 20 degrees of anteversion. This patient was an elderly female, so a 32-mm head with cross-linked polyethylene was used, as opposed to my typical patients who receive a 28-mm femoral head.

Review of surgical reports and especially the implant records is especially important for surgical planning in the patient with recurrent dislocation. We attempt to learn the previous surgical approach, as well as all available liner options for the existing acetabular component, and all existing modular femoral head options for the existing femoral component. If the femoral component is nonmodular, then we determine whether there is a bipolar head available that will fit into the existing acetabular component.

Nonoperative treatment with a brace, hip-girdle strengthening, and precautions are preferred for early postoperative dislocations or patients with medical contraindications to surgery. Early anterior instability is generally felt more amenable to nonoperative treatment, and we ask these patients to sleep with their hip flexed, in hopes that they will heal with a mild flexion contracture. Late dislocations (those with dislocations starting years after surgery), patients who have had multiple recurrent dislocations or multiple previous operations, and patients with weak hip-girdle musculature are more likely to require surgical treatment.

If surgical treatment is necessary, then we take a step-wise approach to the operative procedure. The first step involves choice of the operative approach. Although it is appropriate to choose approach based on surgeon comfort or direction of dislocation, I typically prefer to approach the hip joint through the side where the soft tissues are most deficient. That way one can potentially maintain the intact soft tissues and reduce the risk of global instability. In cases where I do not know the previous approach, I do this by making a short initial incision over the greater trochanter to visualize the abductors. After the old soft tissue defects are recognized, then the incision can be extended into either an anterior side or posterior approach.

A primary goal of every revision for recurrent instability is to optimize implant range of motion. This can be done by reducing impingement, improving implant position, increasing implant length and offset, increasing head size, and increasing soft-tissue tension. As in primary total hip replacement, my goal for hip range of motion is dependent upon the surgical approach taken.

If a posterior approach (with released or deficient posterior soft-tissue but intact anterior soft tissues) has been made, then I shoot for implants that allow greater than 60 degrees of internal rotation in 90 degrees of flexion; with external rotation in full extension that is tethered by the intact anterior soft tissues well before there is impingement and subluxation. If an anterior-side approach has been made, then I shoot for greater than 60 degrees external rotation in full extension; with internal rotation in 90 degrees of flexion that is tethered by the posterior soft tissues well before impingement and subluxation. In cases where there is a complete capsulectomy, or global laxity, I shoot for greater than 60 degrees of rotation with each test.

After the surgical approach is made, the second step in our procedure is to examine the range of motion with the above tests. This step is to confirm the direction of instability, identify sources of impingement, evaluate soft tissue tension, and create goals for improvement in range of motion. An initial assessment of implant position is made as well. After the hip is dislocated, the implant fixation is assessed, and further assessment of implant position is made. If the implants are well fixed and in relatively good position, then the next step is to either remove impingement or trial new femoral heads and acetabular liners.

If the old head and liner are in good condition, then my next step is to eliminate impingement. In general, all nonessential bone and tissue that prevents optimal range of motion is removed. Frequently, for posterior dislocations, there is heterotopic bone in the anterior capsule and gluteus minimus that can be removed. Bony prominences on the anterior greater trochanter and pelvis are removed. Even thickened soft tissue scar can limit range of motion, so this tissue is removed carefully as well.

The next step is to trial new femoral heads and acetabular liners. Either a lateralized acetabular liner or a longer femoral head can improve range of motion by increasing both offset and length. A larger femoral head and liner can increase stability both by improving range of motion and by increasing femoral head "jump distance" prior to dislocation. In addition, a larger femoral head of greater than 36 mm will frequently not have a skirted neck, even at longer neck lengths. Finally an elevated rim acetabular liner is trialed in multiple positions to determine the most resistant to dislocation. While elevated rim liners have been shown to improve stability in revision total hip replacement,[1] it is important to never depend on this technique alone.

In cases where the acetabular component is loose or malpositioned and must be revised, I am prepared to use implants that will accommodate either a large head or constrained liner. If I have to revise the femoral component, then modular femoral components are helpful because both offset and rotation can be adjusted.

Finally, soft tissue tension can be increased by advancement of the greater trochanter or grafting of allograft tissues. I rarely advance the greater trochanter in cases of nonunion that are repairable, and I have no experience at my center with allograft augmentation or other soft tissue tightening techniques.

In cases in which none of the above techniques result in a stable hip, a constrained acetabular liner is considered. One must realize that these devices transfer dislocation forces to implant locking mechanisms and all implant fixation interfaces. Despite that, I have published intermediate-term data suggesting that both the fixation and stability can remain durable at an average of over 10 years with one particular tripolar constraining device (Figure 46-2).[2] The ideal indication for a constrained acetabular component is

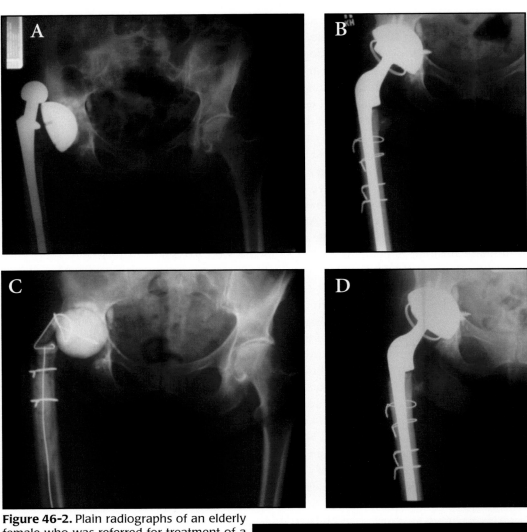

Figure 46-2. Plain radiographs of an elderly female who was referred for treatment of a loose, chronically dislocated, infected, and draining total hip replacement. This patient was treated with a two-stage exchange arthroplasty. The greater trochanter was absent and her abductors were extremely deficient. Because of her extreme soft tissue laxity, her reimplantation was performed with a constrained acetabular component.

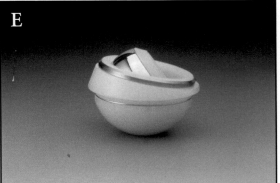

the case where there is extreme soft tissue laxity. These patients are often low demand, elderly, multiply operated, or have abductor insufficiency that cannot be repaired. These patients might have good range of motion in every direction, but severe displacement of the femoral head with the "shuck test." Relative contraindications to use of a constrained liner include implant malposition, persistent impingement, tenuous acetabular fixation, and young active patients.

There are a number of additional important technical considerations when using a constrained acetabular liner: the elevated rim of the liner, if present, should not be positioned where impingement might occur. Large skirted necks should rarely if ever be used with a constrained liner. As many screws as possible should be used to optimally secure the uncemented acetabular shell that will contain a constrained liner. In cases where there is a well-fixed uncemented acetabular shell of sufficient size, the constrained liner can be cemented into the shell.[3] The actual size of the liner should be 2 to 4 mm smaller than the inner diameter of the retained shell, and the liner seated deeply within the shell. If not done by the manufacturer, the polyethylene backside of the liner should be scored with a burr in a spider web pattern. Likewise, if the metal shell is polished or has no holes, it should be scored as well. Also, we usually consider an abduction brace for approximately 6 weeks after any type of revision procedure done for recurrent instability.

References

1. Alberton GM, High WA, Morrey BF. Dislocation after revision total hip arthroplasty: an analysis of risk factors and treatment options. *J Bone Joint Surgery Am.* 2002;84:1788-1792.
2. Goetz DD, Bremner BRB, Callaghan JJ, Capello WN, Johnston RC. Salvage of a recurrently dislocating total hip prosthesis with use of a constrained acetabular component: a concise follow-up of a previous report. *J Bone Joint Surgery Am.* 2004;86:2419-2423.
3. Callaghan JJ, Parvizi J, Novack CC, et al. A constrained liner cemented into a secure cementless acetabular shell. *J Bone Joint Surg Am.* 2004;86:2206-2211.

SECTION X

FAILED

FEMUR QUESTIONS

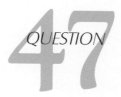
I Have a Patient With a Well-Fixed Extensively Porous-Coated Implant That Needs to Be Removed. How Do I Remove a Well-Fixed Extensively Coated Femoral Component Without Extensive Bone Loss?

Kenneth D. Kleist, MD

As the number of primary and revision total hip arthroplasty procedures has continued to rise, so too has the use of porous-coated acetabular and femoral components. Knowledge of how to remove these components is a critical aspect to revision arthroplasty. In particular, the well-fixed extensively porous-coated femoral component represents a vexing problem to the revision surgeon. Fully coated stems are not only a workhorse revision stem, but are also gaining popularity in primary situations. One must always keep in mind the indications for removing these stems are few and must be carefully considered. The goal of my clinical scenario is consistent with revision surgery in general: minimize bone loss and allow a suitable reconstruction. This requires diligent preoperative planning, appropriate intraoperative tools, and knowledge of how to apply specialized techniques.

Preoperative Evaluation

First, a few clarifications are needed. The most critical part of the process is the preoperative evaluation leading to the decision for revision. We are assuming the appropriate history, physical examination, infectious evaluation, radiographic evaluation, and clinical decision-making process has occurred. A well-fixed stem in this situation means radiographic signs of bone ingrowth or fibrous stability are present using the criteria of Glassman and Engh.[1] An unstable implant, especially an undersized one, is a much different situation. Another important point to keep in mind is that several proximally coated porous stems act as extensively coated implants through distal stem corundum or grit blasting that allows bone ongrowth. This emphasizes the need to know the exact nature and manufacturer of the implants currently in place through previous operative reports or implant records. If unfamiliar with the stem, I ask the manufacturer representative for information that will lay out its geometry and areas of porous surface. This knowledge is critical to avoiding unexpected problems in the operating room.

Templating

Extended trochanteric osteotomy (ETO) with sectioning of the femoral stem for removal of these implants is well established.[2,3] Alternative options have been proposed, including episiotomy of the femur and cortical slots or windows. While many of these techniques have been successful in experienced hands, they do not provide the visualization, access, speed, or control of an ETO, especially if acetabular access is needed. It also provides inline neutral access to the femoral isthmus for ease of preparation of the femoral reconstruction. Studies indicate reliable ETO healing even in the face of infection.[4] Preoperatively, the exact length of the osteotomy must be planned. An appropriate anterior-posterior (AP) pelvis, AP, and lateral of the hip are needed. With a significant portion of the femur visible, I template the ETO to the level where the stem becomes cylindrical, or rarely a short stem allows osteotomy to the tip of the stem with enough remaining isthmus for stable fixation. In a long-bowed stem the osteotomy should go to the level of the maximal bow. The same applies if a significant proximal femoral varus deformity exists. Ideally, 4 to 5 cm of intact isthmus is left for fixation of the next stem.

Tools

A set of hollow core trephines must be available in small increments up to at least 0.5 mm greater than the size of the implant (Figure 47-1). A universal extractor and any specialized removal tools for the implant you are working with are helpful. A high-speed drill with pencil tip burrs and tungsten carbide metal cutting burrs or discs are needed. Multiple tungsten carbide burrs may be needed to section the stem. Also needed are oscillating saws, a Gigli saw, flexible osteotomes of various sizes and lengths, broad osteotomes, Bennett retractors, and fixation for the osteotomy. In femurs with poor proximal bone stock, you may wish to have strut allograft and greater trochanteric fixation plates available to provide additional support.

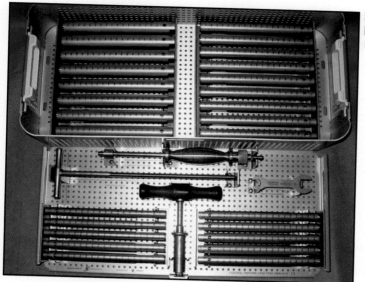

Figure 47-1. A complete set of hollow trephines is needed.

Operative Technique

Intraoperatively, a posterior approach is performed. Any remaining short external rotators are removed from the trochanter and the pseudocapsule is excised with appropriate cell count, cultures, and frozen sections sent. The distal extent of the exposure is determined by preoperative templating. Once exposed, I like to mark the path of my osteotomy with the electrocautery along the posterior aspect of the femur. I usually take one-third of the femoral circumference, leaving as much of the gluteus maximus attachment intact on the main femoral piece. I then use a pencil tip burr to start the distal aspect of the osteotomy first. I round the distal corners and start back up anteriorly 1 to 2 cm. In a similar fashion, make sure the anterior soft tissue is released from the proximal and anterior trochanter region. The osteotomy is then initiated proximally and anteriorly as well. This helps to prevent uncontrolled osteotomy fragment fracture. I then use an oscillating saw to cut to the level of the prosthesis posteriorly. Alternatively, a microsagittal saw or multiple drill holes connected with osteotomes may be used. Carefully, several broad osteotomes are used to pry the fragment off the implant until it cracks anteriorly. Bennett retractors are then used to protect the osteotomy fragment anteriorly. You are now staring at the lateral shoulder of the prosthesis. Remember, studies have shown that ingrowth along fully porous stem tends to occur along the entire prosthesis, not just distally. All interfaces will need to be disrupted. Anteriorly and posteriorly, a pencil tip burr or flexible osteotomes can be used to disrupt the interfaces. A Gigli saw is then used to disrupt the medial interface. Multiple passes and saws may be required. Once these accessible interfaces are disrupted, the universal extractor is attached and 3 firm removal attempts are made. If the stem does not move at all, it must be sectioned and removed with trephines.

A metal-cutting disc or burr is used with the high-speed drill. Soft tissues are protected from debris with laparotomy sponges and irrigation is used. The stem is cut at the distal extent of the osteotomy and must be in the cylindrical portion. The proximal body is then removed. A hollow trephine of 0.5 mm larger than the known size of the stem is used with copious irrigation to ream over the stem. Fluoroscopy can be used for this portion, but usually you can tell by your advancement and the amount of metal debris whether you are angling off course. Ultimately, when the last interface is disrupted, the stem often incarcerates in the trephine and is removed with the trephine. The femur is then reconstructed in the appropriate fashion, or an antibiotic spacer is inserted. Repair of the osteotomy is done using 2 to 3 cables or alternatively Luque wires. Luque wires are my fixation of choice in infection because of the lack of braided material. Postoperatively, active abduction is restricted for 6 weeks to allow adequate healing of the osteotomy. Most people also advocate a period of protected weight bearing as well.

References

1. Glassman AH, Engh CA. The removal of porous-coated femoral hip stems. *Clin Orthop Relat Res.* 1992;285: 164-180.
2. Paprosky WG, Weeden SH, Bowling JW. Component removal in revision total hip arthroplasty. *Clin Orthop Relat Res.* 2001;393:181-193.
3. Masri BA, Mitchell PA, Duncan CP. Removal of solidly fixed implants during revision hip and knee arthroplasty. *J Am Acad Orthop Surg.* 2005;13(1):18-27.
4. Morshed S, Huffman GR, Ries MD. Extended trochanteric osteotomy for 2-stage revision for infected total hip arthroplasty. *J Arthroplasty.* 2005;20(3):294-301.

A Patient Fell and Now Has a Periprosthetic Femur Fracture With a Loose Femoral Component. How Should I Approach This Surgery?

Tad L. Gerlinger, MD

The Vancouver classification categorizes periprosthetic fractures about a hip arthroplasty according to the site of the fracture, the stability of the implant, and the integrity of the surrounding bone stock.[1] Fracture location dictates the type: A, proximal to the prosthesis; B, including or just below the prosthesis; and C, well below the stem tip. Subtypes are labeled 1 for a stable prosthesis and 2 for an unstable prosthesis. If bone stock is compromised by osteopenia, osteolysis, or severe comminution, then subtype 3 applies. This classification system is both reliable and valid when used by experts and nonexperts.[1] The greatest value of this classification system is that it guides treatment decisions that will optimize outcome.

The authors based the classification on 4 critical questions that the surgeon should answer before making a treatment decision. Does the fracture involve the prosthesis? Is the fracture unstable? Is the component loose? Is bone stock adequate? Once these questions have been answered, a decision to fix the fracture without revision of components, revise the components and fix the fracture, or revise the components and augment bone stock can be made.

For a fracture proximal to a stable prosthesis, the fracture may be addressed in isolation. These Type A fractures involve the greater or lesser trochanters. Greater trochanteric fractures may be fixed with a claw-type device, cables, or cerclage wires if unstable and lesser trochanteric fractures can generally be treated expectantly with activity modification. A decision for fixation is made when abductor function or hip stability are in question.

A useful tool for fractures distal to a well-fixed stem, Type C fractures, is the cable plate. This device allows cable fixation proximal to the tip of the stem and screw fixation distal. There are biomechanical data supporting unicortical screws proximal as well. I

Figure 48-1. Type B2 fracture.

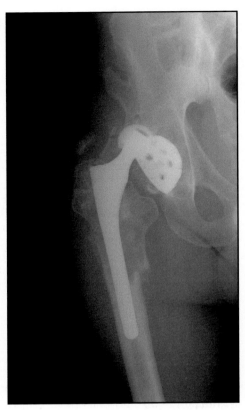

advocate 8 cortices of distal screw fixation with a 4.5 mm or equivalent caliber plate and an equivalent number of cables and unicortical screws proximally to ensure rigid fixation. Comminution or instability of the fracture pattern may dictate a longer device with more fixation. A long fixed-angle device with purchase into the femoral condyles may be necessary for long oblique or very distal fractures. Care should be taken to ensure that the plate and the stem overlap to eliminate stress risers. There is also recent literature supporting indirect reduction and use of percutaneous plating.

The case pictured (Figure 48-1) represents a Type B2, a fracture at the level of a loose femoral component. It is an unstable fracture and bone stock is marginal proximal to the fracture, but adequate distally. The femoral component must be revised, stem fixation obtained distally, and the fracture stabilized. The femoral component revision classification of Paprosky[2] is useful in evaluating the feasibility of using a porous fully coated implant in the treatment of Type B fractures. Paprosky Type I femurs have minimal metaphyseal defects with an intact diaphysis. Type II is characterized by major metaphyseal bone loss with an intact diaphysis. Type IIIA femurs have defects that extend to the junction of the metaphysis and diaphysis and Type IIIB is characterized by diaphyseal deficiency with maintenance of at least 4 cm of diaphysis distal to the isthmus. Type IV femurs have essentially no diaphyseal bone in which to obtain purchase with an uncemented stem. Using this classification, all but Type IV femurs may support a porous-coated implant. Addressing the bone distal to the fracture will provide stable implant

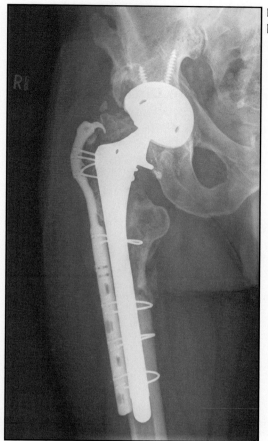

Figure 48-2. Type B2 fracture treated with a fully porous coated stem and trochanteric plate.

fixation without relying on fracture fixation and is my technique of choice for Type B2 periprosthetic fractures.

I prefer an extensile posterior approach to these fractures. Many times the fracture will provide access to the proximal aspect of the stem. An extended trochanteric osteotomy is a good option for a cemented prosthesis to allow easy cement removal. I recommend performing cement removal as late in the case as possible to "protect" the greater trochanteric bone. If the prosthesis is uncemented, it is sometimes possible to preserve the proximal femur as a sleeve, through which the diaphyseal femur is prepared. A cable placed around the proximal intact diaphysis of the femur will lessen your risk of fracture during reaming. I recommend under-reaming by 0.5 mm for the 4 cm of "scratch fit" on which the porous implant relies for fixation. This is easily checked by inserting the prosthesis by hand and ensuring that you can advance it within 4.5 to 5 cm of its final position. Caution should be used when stem size is greater than 19 mm in Paprosky Type IIIB femurs, as a high failure rate has been reported.[3] After obtaining stable distal prosthesis fixation, the proximal femur can be secured with cerclage wires, cables, or trochanteric claw-type plates, with or without strut grafts (Figure 48-2). In elderly patients, those with overall poor bone quality, and Paprosky Type IV femurs, a cemented tumor prosthesis with or without proximal femoral replacement should be considered.

Type B1 fractures should be evaluated cautiously. Although several authors report success with fixing the fracture in isolation, determining the stability of the stem can be difficult. The most prudent approach is to assume that the prosthesis is loose and proceed as for a Type B2. If the stem is indeed well fixed, then the fracture can undergo open reduction internal fixation as for a Type C.

By asking the 4 questions advocated by the authors of the Vancouver classification, a plan for treatment of a periprosthetic hip fracture can be formulated. Evaluating the femoral bone quality according to the Paprosky classification will predict success in obtaining distal fixation with a revision fully porous-coated stem. A porous fully coated stem allows you to bypass the fracture and is my implant of choice for a periprosthetic hip fracture with a loose stem.

References

1. Brady O, Garbuz D, Masri B, et al. Classification of the hip. *Orthop Clin North Am*. 1999;30:215-220.
2. Paprosky W, Bradford M, Younger T. Classification of bone defects in failed prosthesis. *Chir Organi Mov*. 1994;79(4):285-291.
3. Sporer S, Paprosky W. Revision total hip arthroplasty: the limits of fully coated stems. *Clin Orthop Relat Res*. 2003;417:203-209.

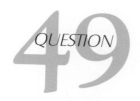

A Patient Fell and Now Has a Periprosthetic Femur Fracture With a Well-Fixed Femoral Component. How Should I Approach This Surgery?

Mark Dumonski, MD
Walter W. Virkus, MD

We are seeing periprosthetic fractures around a total hip arthroplasty (THA) more frequently. In a report of over 30,000 THAs, the incidence of femoral periprosthetic fracture was found to be 1.1% following primary THA and 4% after revisions.[1] An increased risk of periprosthetic hip fracture is associated with oversized femoral components, motion of loose components, osteolysis, and removal of previously placed hardware. Patients with neurologic disorders and osteoporosis are also at increased risk of fracture. While the majority of periprosthetic femur fractures occur postoperatively, intraoperative fractures also occur. These are usually during hip dislocation or implantation of press-fit stems.

We use the Vancouver classification system in characterizing femoral periprosthetic hip fractures (Figure 49-1).[2] It is helpful in that it guides treatment. Type A fractures are proximal to the distal tip of the stem and are subcategorized as involving either the greater trochanter (A_G) or the lesser trochanter (A_L). These are again subdivided into stable or unstable fractures. Type B fractures occur in the area of the distal stem. These are subcategorized as having a femoral component that is well fixed (B1), loose (B2), or loose with inadequate bone stock (B3). Type C fractures are distal to the stem.

Most femoral periprosthetic fractures around a THA require operative intervention, the exception being incomplete longitudinal proximal fractures only noticed postoperatively (occurring during or after surgery). In this situation, weight bearing should be protected and radiographs should be followed closely. We treat unstable Vancouver A fractures of the greater trochanter with cerclage cables in conjunction with a claw device to improve stability of the fracture fragment. For Vancouver B1 fractures, we prefer plate and screw fixation supplemented with cerclage wires proximally if necessary. Locking

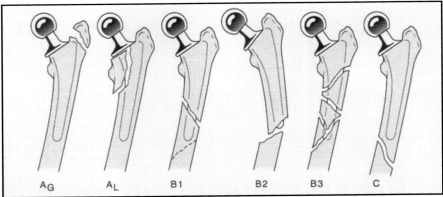

Figure 49-1. Vancouver classification for periprosthetic femoral fractures. (Reprinted from Berry DJ. Epidemiology: hip and knee. In: Duncan C, Callaghan J, eds. *Periprosthetic Fractures After Major Joint Replacement.* Philadelphia, PA: WB Saunders; 1999:183-190.)

plates are very useful when plating these fractures.[3,4] Short locking screws are available and can be placed into the femoral cortex around the THA stem or even into the cement mantle. Additionally, we are often able to place longer standard screws aimed anterior or posterior that miss the THA stem or glance off it. These screws give excellent proximal purchase. We have not had any problems with breakage of the cement mantle or damage to the THA stem. Occasionally, we add 1 or 2 cerclage wires if we feel additional proximal plate/bone fixation is required, but it is important to keep the cerclage wires as far from the fracture site as possible to minimize compromising the blood supply. In fractures with a single fracture line, the decision must be made whether to achieve anatomic reduction, which is then stabilized with a lag screw and plate, or nonanatomic reduction, which focuses on length, alignment, and rotation, which is stabilized with plate without a lag screw (Figure 49-2). In the setting of significant comminution, anatomic reduction should be avoided as it is associated with extensive soft tissue stripping and increases the likelihood of nonunion. Proper limb length, alignment, and rotation are the goal in these cases, with fracture stabilization being achieved with a plate spanning the fracture comminution (bridge plating). Rotational alignment is best evaluated by clinical inspection of the patella and comparing this relationship to the uninjured contralateral extremity. Length is best assessed by measuring the distance from the anterior superior iliac spine to the medial malleolus on the injured and contralateral extremity. We find the electrocautery cord to be useful for this measurement. We avoid allograft struts in these cases unless there is significant thinning of the cortices or large osseous shaft defects, which is rare. We feel that the healing the allograft to the host femur is highly variable, and that the devascularization of the fracture area necessary for their placement significantly hinders the healing of the fracture.

Type B2 fractures require removal of the loose prosthesis and a long femoral stem revision supplemented cerclage fixation of the proximal fracture. B3 fractures must be treated with an allograft-prosthetic composite, a tumor prosthesis, or an uncemented long-stem revision. Type C fractures can generally be treated independent of the prosthesis, using plating techniques similar to those described for B1 fractures. We avoid short retrograde

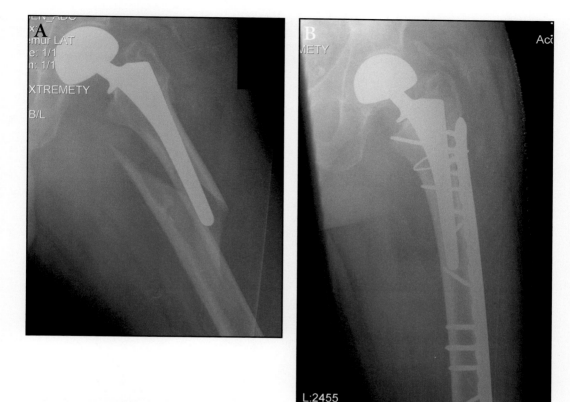

Figure 49-2. (A) AP radiograph of an 88-year-old male with a type B1 periprosthetic femur fracture. (B) Postoperative AP radiograph demonstrates anatomic fixation with a plate and screw construct supplemented with a cable proximally.

nails even when theoretically feasible because of the stress risers they create between the nail and the tip of the THA stem.

Conclusion

Management of fractures around a THA is determined by the stability of the stem. Unstable stems require revision, and fracture management in these cases typically centers around "recreating the tube" to facilitate revision arthroplasty. Fractures with stable stems are treated with open reduction, internal fixation using techniques that minimize compromising the vascular environment of the fracture.

References

1. Berry DJ. Epidemiology: hip and knee. In: Duncan C, Callaghan J, eds. *Periprosthetic Fractures After Major Joint Replacement*. Philadelphia, PA: WB Saunders; 1999:183-190.
2. Duncan C, Masri B. Fractures of the femur after hip replacement. *Inst Course Lect.* 1995;44:293-304.

3. Tsiridis ET, Narvani AA, Timperley JA, Gie GA. Dynamic compression plates for Vancouver type B periprosthetic femoral fractures: a 3-year follow-up of 18 cases. *Acta Orthop.* 2005;76:531-537.
4. Ricci WM, Bolhofner BR, Loftus T, Cox C, Mitchell S, Borrelli J. Indirect reduction and plate fixation with grafting, for periprosthetic femoral shaft fractures about a stable intramedullary implant. *J Bone Joint Surg Am.* 2005;87:2240-2245.

INDEX

Printed in the United States
by Baker & Taylor Publisher Services